Cradled in Light

Navigating Love and Loss in the
Neonatal Intensive Care Unit

Arwin M. Valencia, MD, FAAP

Copyright Notice

Table of Contents

Dedicated to the parents, families, and caregivers who have loved beyond measure and grieved beyond words.

Cradled in Light

In the stillness where breath meets dawn,
A fragile miracle is gently drawn.
You held a universe in your hands,
Love unspoken, yet it understands.

For even the briefest spark burns bright,
A soul now cradled in holy light.
Amid the hum of hope and care,
You whispered prayers into the sterile air.

Each heartbeat echoed love's refrain,
Each touch a balm for joy and pain.
Through tears and tremors, faith took flight
You kept the vigil of sacred light.

Though moments passed like falling stars,
They left their mark upon your scars.
For love unmeasured cannot fade,
Nor by time or sorrow be unmade.

Your child, your heart, your guiding light,
Still glows beyond the veil of night.
In grief's embrace, you learned to feel,
That love transcends, that time can heal.

The cradle may now stand alone,
Yet light remains, it has not flown.
For every sigh and every tear,
Love whispers softly: I am here.

So, lift your gaze where heaven gleams,
Your baby rests within your dreams.
No distance, death, nor shadowed way,
Can dim the dawn of love's new day.

Their soul lives on, pure, infinite, bright,
Forever cradled in eternal light.

Foreword

by

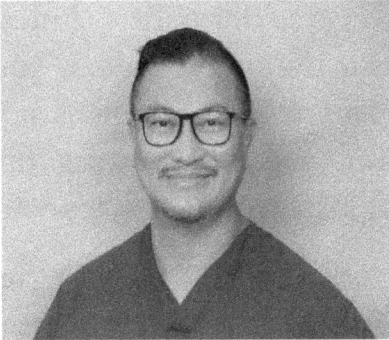

Arwin M. Valencia, MD FAAP

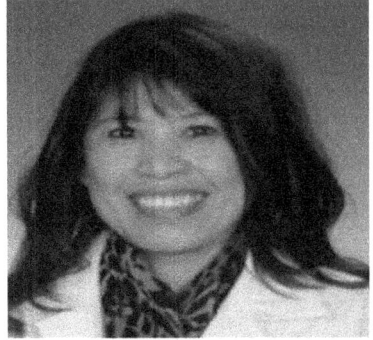

Maria A. Abrantes, MD FAAP

Arwin M. Valencia, MD and Maria A. Abrantes, MD,
board-certified neonatologists whose careers have been dedicated
to caring for the most fragile beginnings of life.

In the delicate world of neonatal medicine, where life often begins in fragile balance, compassion is not an accessory to clinical excellence, it is its very foundation. The neonatal intensive care unit (NICU) stands as both a sanctuary of science and a crucible of emotion, where the smallest lives fight the greatest battles, and where parents experience the profound tension between hope and fear. Within these walls, compassionate neonatal care emerges not merely as a philosophy but as a necessity—an approach that bridges science and humanity, healing and faith, precision and presence.

The Heart of Compassionate Neonatal Care

Compassionate neonatal care is a holistic practice that weaves medical expertise with emotional sensitivity and spiritual awareness. It recognizes that every infant, regardless of size or gestational age, is not only a clinical patient but also a person whose dignity, comfort, and connection matter deeply. Similarly, every parent is not just a caregiver but a partner in healing—bearing the invisible wounds of uncertainty, exhaustion, and hope.

The compassionate approach seeks to address both the physiological needs of the newborn and the psychological and spiritual needs of the family. It is guided by one central truth: **healing begins where understanding and empathy meet.**

Family-centered care, the cornerstone of compassionate neonatal medicine, empowers parents to participate actively in their child's journey. The *Compassionate Family Care Framework (CFCF)* advocates for this partnership, ensuring that parents do not feel like passive observers in the care of their child but rather integral members of the team. Allowing limitless parental presence in the NICU, involving them in daily decisions, and respecting their intuition as parents cultivate not only trust but also resilience.

This empowerment transforms fear into purpose. When parents are invited to hold, feed, or comfort their infant, even in the midst of critical care, a sacred connection is strengthened. These moments, small yet profound, become the emotional scaffolding that helps families endure the storms of uncertainty.

Principles That Shape Compassionate Practice

The principles of compassionate neonatal care extend beyond clinical routines; they form a moral and emotional compass for caregivers.

1.   Open and Honest Communication.

Transparency builds trust. Families deserve clear, timely, and empathetic communication about their baby's condition, prognosis, and treatment options. Difficult conversations, when handled with sincerity and kindness, create space for shared understanding rather than despair. The goal is not merely to deliver information, but to *accompany* families through it.

2.   Parental Presence and Involvement.

Limitless parental access honors the natural bond between infant and parent. Studies have shown that skin-to-skin contact, known as *kangaroo care*, stabilizes heart rate, improves oxygenation, and promotes weight gain. Yet its emotional benefit is even greater—it reassures both baby and parent that they are not alone.

3.   **Focus on Comfort and Healing.**

Programs such as the *Neonatal Comfort Care Program (NCCP)* remind us that medicine is not always about cure, but always about care. From diagnosis through the transition home—or, in heartbreaking cases, through the end of life—comfort remains the guiding light. Pain management, gentle touch, soothing voices, and individualized attention all reinforce the message that even in suffering, dignity is preserved.

4.   **Holistic Support.**

The NICU environment can be overwhelming, with its constant alarms, machines, and emotional intensity. A holistic model acknowledges the mental and social dimensions of healing. Social workers, psychologists, chaplains, and peer-to-peer parent support groups become integral members of the care team, helping families navigate fear, guilt, and grief.

5.   **Celebrating Milestones.**

Every gram gained, every breath taken without assistance, every day of stability is a triumph worth honoring. Marking these milestones brings light into a setting often shrouded in worry. The celebration of small victories reminds families—and staff alike—that progress, however incremental, is sacred.

6.   **Supporting Families with Unique Challenges.**
Compassionate care is not one-size-fits-all. Families facing neonatal opioid withdrawal, congenital anomalies, or end-of-life decisions require specialized support that balances clinical precision with deep respect for their emotional and ethical struggles. The role of the healthcare team is not to judge but to walk alongside, ensuring access to resources, counseling, and unconditional compassion.

7.   **Clinical Empathy.**

Compassion in medicine is not sentimentality—it is a disciplined form of understanding. Clinical empathy demands that healthcare professionals truly *see* the infant and family before them, listening with both intellect and heart. This dual awareness enriches medical judgment and fortifies the bond between healer and patient.

The Benefits of Compassionate Care

When compassion infuses the clinical environment, measurable benefits unfold.

For infants, symptom management becomes more effective, leading to reduced stress and pain. Gentle handling, reduced noise exposure, and family presence all contribute to better physiologic stability. For parents, compassionate engagement decreases anxiety, fosters confidence, and strengthens coping mechanisms. They leave the NICU not only with a healed baby but with restored faith in themselves as caregivers.

For healthcare providers, compassion brings coherence and meaning to their work. The emotional toll of witnessing suffering can lead to burnout, yet compassion, when nurtured collectively, becomes a source of resilience. In environments where empathy and teamwork are valued, staff experience higher morale and a renewed sense of purpose.

The Integration of Science, Humanity, and Faith in Medicine

Modern medicine stands at a remarkable intersection—an age where technology allows us to sustain life in ways unimaginable just decades ago. Yet, as machines grow more precise, there arises a deeper need to preserve the soul of care. To heal fully, we must integrate the triad of **science, humanity, and faith.**

Science: The Foundation of Healing

Science is the anchor upon which neonatal medicine rests. Evidence-based practice, rigorous research, and technological innovation have transformed survival outcomes for preterm and critically ill infants. Ventilators, incubators, surfactant therapy, and advanced imaging have become lifelines for the tiniest patients.

Scientific inquiry ensures that interventions are safe, effective, and continually refined. It offers the data that guide our hands and inform our minds. Yet, as powerful as science is, it cannot alone touch the heart of suffering. The physician who knows the latest research but not the tears of a grieving parent practices medicine only in part.

Humanity: The Art of Healing

The humanities remind us that medicine is not merely a science of the body but a ministry to the soul. Narrative medicine, ethics, and communication studies re-center the patient as a whole being—biological, emotional, and existential. Through storytelling, reflection, and empathy training, healthcare professionals cultivate the sensitivity needed to interpret not only laboratory results but also the unspoken language of pain and hope.

Humanity in medicine is what transforms treatment into healing. It compels the clinician to pause amid procedures, to notice the trembling hand of a mother, to explain a diagnosis with gentleness, to grieve alongside the family when loss becomes inevitable.

For providers themselves, engaging with the humanities is restorative. Art, music, literature, and reflective writing offer spaces for processing grief and preventing compassion fatigue. They remind caregivers that before they were clinicians, they were human beings—capable of wonder, sorrow, and grace.

Faith: The Spirit of Healing

For many families, faith becomes the lifeline that sustains them when medical certainty falls short. Whether rooted in organized religion or personal spirituality, faith offers meaning amid chaos. To a parent praying over a fragile newborn, faith becomes a language beyond statistics—a dialogue with the divine that transcends outcomes.

Acknowledging this dimension in the NICU does not blur professional boundaries; rather, it affirms the patient's wholeness. When healthcare providers recognize the sacredness of life and the mystery that accompanies it, their care gains depth. Faith may also serve as a moral compass for clinicians, anchoring them in humility and ethical integrity.

Spiritual care teams, including chaplains and counselors, play an essential role in integrating faith within the healthcare setting. Their presence complements the physician's role, creating a space where families can voice their fears, doubts, and hopes. Research continues to show that patients who feel spiritually supported report higher satisfaction, greater emotional resilience, and even improved physiological recovery.

Ethical Integration: The Balance of the Three Pillars

The challenge and beauty of integrating science, humanity, and faith lie in maintaining balance. No single pillar should overshadow the others; instead, they should coexist in harmony, informing one another.

For healthcare providers, this means practicing evidence-based medicine with a heart attuned to empathy and a spirit grounded in humility. Respecting patient autonomy remains paramount—faith discussions must always be patient-led and consent-based. Taking a brief *spiritual history* during admission allows clinicians to understand whether and how a patient's beliefs influence care preferences. When needed, collaboration with chaplains or spiritual care providers ensures that the infant and family receive holistic support.

For medical institutions, integration calls for structural and educational initiatives. Medical schools increasingly embed humanities courses into their curricula, training future physicians not only in anatomy and pharmacology but also in compassion and communication. Hospitals can further this mission through faith-informed outreach programs, community health education, and culturally sensitive care models.

For families and society, the integration of these three forces offers reassurance that medicine remains a human endeavor. When science upholds evidence, humanity upholds empathy, and faith upholds meaning, care becomes complete.

A Call to Compassionate Renewal

In the rapidly evolving landscape of healthcare, it is tempting to let efficiency, data, and technology dominate the conversation. Yet, the soul of medicine still resides in presence—in the quiet moments when a nurse hums a lullaby to a premature infant, when a physician kneels beside grieving parents, or when a chaplain prays softly in the background as life and death dance their fragile waltz.

Compassionate neonatal care invites us to remember that behind every monitor is a miracle in progress, behind every statistic a story of love, and behind every medical professional a human being striving to honor the sanctity of life. The call, therefore, is not only to heal the infant but to hold the family, to educate with empathy, and to practice medicine as both art and ministry.

As we look to the future of neonatal care, let it be one where science continues to innovate, humanity continues to soften, and faith continues to inspire. For it is at this intersection—where knowledge meets kindness and where healing meets holiness—that true medicine is born.

Introduction:
Cradled Between Worlds

The Neonatal Intensive Care Unit (NICU) stands as one of the most paradoxical places in medicine, a space where the precision of science meets the mystery of the soul. It is at once a center of advanced technological innovation and a sacred sanctuary where the rawest human emotions, hope, fear, love, and surrender, are laid bare. Within its walls, the boundaries between medicine, ethics, and spirituality blur, revealing the profound complexity of what it means to preserve life at its most fragile beginning.

The NICU as a Scientific Frontier

The NICU embodies the pinnacle of modern medicine. It is both a laboratory of progress and a battlefield for survival, where the tiniest patients depend on extraordinary innovation to bridge the gap between viability and vitality.

Advanced Technology and Equipment

Every piece of equipment in the NICU tells a story of decades of research and relentless pursuit of progress. High-frequency ventilators deliver hundreds of micro-breaths per minute—small, precise puffs that protect delicate lungs still learning to breathe the world's air. Non-invasive monitors, guided by artificial intelligence, record oxygen levels, brain activity, and heart rhythms with astonishing accuracy, reducing physical disturbance and allowing infants to rest undisturbed in their incubators.

Recent developments in *artificial womb* technology—like the experimental "Biobag"—seek to mimic the maternal environment, potentially allowing extremely premature infants to continue growing in an extrauterine yet fluid-filled world. Such innovation hints at a future where survival at the threshold of life may no longer be the exception but the expectation. Similarly, breakthroughs in surfactant therapy, neuroprotective hypothermia, and personalized nutrition programs have redefined neonatal survival, transforming outcomes once deemed impossible into daily realities.

Medical Research and Innovation

The NICU is also a living laboratory of discovery. Artificial intelligence helps clinicians anticipate complications before they manifest, using vast datasets to tailor treatment plans for each infant's unique physiology. Genetic research explores the potential of correcting congenital conditions in utero or through targeted postnatal therapy. Stem cell research, once confined to theoretical discussion, now moves closer to repairing damaged organs—lungs scarred by oxygen toxicity or brains injured by hypoxia.

Even bedside ultrasound—a quiet, non-invasive tool—has revolutionized neonatal diagnostics. With a probe the size of a pen, physicians can visualize the infant's heart, brain, or abdomen within seconds, eliminating the need for stressful transport to distant imaging suites. These innovations together create an ecosystem of healing where science extends the reach of compassion.

The NICU as a Sacred Space

While technology forms the backbone of the NICU, its heart beats with something beyond the measurable. It is, for many families, a *temple of vulnerability and hope*, where life's mysteries are contemplated as deeply as its mechanisms are studied.

A Place of Spiritual Significance

Parents entering the NICU step into a realm where time stands still. Machines hum rhythmically, monitors pulse softly, and the air feels heavy with anticipation. Here, faith—whether religious, spiritual, or simply rooted in love—becomes both anchor and compass.

Many families find themselves sanctifying their child's struggle, interpreting each day as a sacred encounter with the divine. Theologians call this "spiritual coping"—a way to derive meaning amidst chaos. For some, it manifests as whispered prayers, for others, as gratitude for each heartbeat on the monitor. Hospitals that integrate spiritual care teams recognize the immense value of this dimension.

Chaplains walk beside families through moments of despair and grace alike, often guiding rituals that honor cultural or religious practices. At Stanford Children's Health, for example, families fold origami cranes—symbols of hope and healing—each one a prayer embodied in paper.

Even in the shadow of loss, the NICU becomes a chapel of remembrance. In end-of-life care, spiritual presence helps families navigate grief not as defeat, but as a sacred transformation—a return of their child's spirit to its source.

The Intimacy of Family-Centered Care

Family-centered care has become the gold standard in neonatal medicine, emphasizing that parents are not mere observers but essential partners. The practice of *kangaroo care*—skin-to-skin contact between parent and infant—transcends the boundaries of science, awakening something primal and sacred. These moments, often accompanied by tears and gratitude, strengthen the baby's heart rate, oxygenation, and emotional stability, while healing the parents' fear and helplessness.

The relationship between families and caregivers in the NICU often evolves into one of profound mutual trust. Nurses, in particular, serve as both healers and emotional anchors. They witness the daily triumphs and heartbreaks, offering not only medical expertise but human tenderness. For parents, these caregivers often become surrogate family, their presence a reminder that they are not alone in this sacred vigil.

The Ethical Dimensions of a Dual Role

The NICU's dual identity—as both a technological frontier and a sanctuary of humanity—inevitably invites profound ethical reflection. Each decision to intervene, prolong, or withdraw care sits at the crossroads of science, morality, and compassion.

Balancing Treatment and Suffering

As technology advances, the question of "Can we?" must be tempered with "Should we?" The capacity to sustain life through invasive means brings the ethical obligation to consider the quality of that life. Clinicians face the agonizing task of balancing aggressive treatment with the imperative to minimize suffering. Each act of resuscitation carries not only physical implications but moral and spiritual ones.

Shared Decision-Making

In neonatology, the principle of autonomy is uniquely complex. The patient cannot speak; thus, parents become the voice of the infant's best interest. But their voices are often strained under the weight of hope, guilt, and uncertainty. Physicians must navigate these emotional currents with humility, ensuring decisions are made through shared understanding rather than paternal authority. True compassion lies not in dictating outcomes but in co-authoring them with empathy and respect.

Access and Equity

Ethical reflection also extends beyond the bedside to the societal realm. Cutting-edge technology, though miraculous, risks deepening inequities if access depends on geography or wealth. The challenge for modern neonatology is not only to innovate but to democratize innovation—to ensure that every child, regardless of circumstance, can benefit from humanity's progress.

The Paradox of Control and Surrender

At its core, the NICU embodies the paradox of the modern human condition: the simultaneous drive to *control life* and the spiritual call to *surrender to its mystery*. The very technologies designed to protect life also confront us with the humbling truth of our limitations.

The Technological Impulse: Control and Comfort

Humanity's march toward mastery over nature has yielded extraordinary results. We have doubled our lifespan, cured diseases, and extended the boundaries of survival. Yet this same impulse—to predict, prevent, and perfect—can distance us from life's deeper lessons.

Technology promises control, but in doing so, it tempts us with the illusion of invincibility. Our gadgets, algorithms, and artificial intelligences give the impression that uncertainty is a flaw to be engineered out of existence. But the NICU reminds us that control is never absolute. A single heartbeat, a fragile breath, can shatter the illusion and return us to the humility of being.

The Spiritual Significance of Fragility

Paradoxically, it is in our most fragile moments that we encounter the sacred. The recognition of life's impermanence infuses each moment with value. Spiritual traditions across cultures affirm that suffering and limitation are not punishments, but pathways to growth, gratitude, and grace.

Surrender, therefore, is not defeat—it is alignment. To surrender is to acknowledge that while science serves life, it does not own it. In embracing fragility, we open the door to resilience, compassion, and connection. It is the awareness of mortality that transforms medicine from a mechanical trade into a ministry of love.

The Emerging Paradox: Progress and Presence

The coexistence of technological mastery and spiritual vulnerability creates a profound tension in modern care.

If the pursuit of longevity becomes the sole objective, medicine risks becoming dehumanized—focused more on metrics than meaning. A life prolonged without presence, purpose, or peace may achieve quantity but lose quality.

Likewise, a society obsessed with perfection may forget the sanctity of imperfection, where empathy and compassion are born.

The NICU forces us to confront this paradox directly. It is a place where data and devotion coexist, where machines sustain the rhythm of life but cannot measure the pulse of love. Amidst the alarms and monitors, a silent question lingers: *Is the goal to extend life at all costs, or to honor life in all its forms, even when it fades?*

A Neonatologist's Reflection: Between Action and Surrender

For me, neonatology is not merely a profession—it is a vocation, a sacred calling to honor life itself. Each time I enter the NICU, I am reminded that I stand at the threshold between two worlds: the scientific and the spiritual, the tangible and the transcendent.

To resuscitate a newborn is to witness creation in its rawest form—to hold in one's hands the fragile spark of being. The urgency to restore that first breath can become overwhelming, driven by the desire to conquer death. Yet, when efforts fail, the ensuing grief and self-blame reveal an important truth: that not all outcomes are ours to control. There lies a subtle danger when success or failure in resuscitation becomes a reflection of ego rather than compassion.

Over the years, I have come to understand that medicine, at its highest form, is not about victory—it is about reverence. It is about acting with precision and surrendering with grace. To know when to fight and when to let go is perhaps the greatest wisdom any healer can cultivate.

This understanding has shaped my motivation for writing this work. It is a call to balance—between science and soul, between effort and acceptance. It is a reminder that we are instruments, not architects, of destiny. Our duty is to serve life, to honor its fragility, and to act always with love and humility. For every infant we touch carries not only the promise of biology, but the essence of the divine.

Conclusion: The NICU as a Mirror of Humanity

In the end, the Neonatal Intensive Care Unit is more than a medical environment—it is a mirror reflecting the human condition. It reveals our capacity for innovation and compassion, our yearning for control, and our ultimate need for surrender. It is where science kneels before mystery and where caregivers learn that healing is not always synonymous with curing.

The NICU reminds us that life's fragility is not its flaw, it is its greatest gift. For in our shared vulnerability lies the source of our deepest strength, our truest compassion, and our most profound understanding of love.

PART I

Foundations of Life and Loss in the NICU

Chapter 1 – The Science of Beginnings
The Fragile Transition to Life

There are no moments more breathtaking than the first breath of a newborn. In that instant, the silence of the womb gives way to the cry of life—a sound so small, yet it reverberates across eternity. I have witnessed that moment countless times, yet it never ceases to stir something ancient within me. It is the sound of creation replaying itself, the sacred choreography of spirit entering flesh.

As a neonatologist, I live at the intersection where science and divinity meet—where physiology becomes poetry, and the ordinary act of breathing becomes a miracle. The transition from womb to world is a masterwork of design, a fragile balancing act between dependency and autonomy. It is a biological revolution that takes place in mere seconds, and when it falters, we—the guardians of beginnings—step in to guide life across that narrow bridge.

Inside the womb, a baby floats in the warmth of amniotic waters, sustained by the steady rhythm of a mother's heart. Oxygen comes not through lungs, but through the whispering currents of the placenta. The fetal heart beats with purpose, yet its path is unlike ours; it flows through secret doorways—shunts that bypass the lungs, for air is not yet the medium of life.

Then, with birth, everything changes. The cord is clamped. The lungs fill. The heart reroutes its flow. And the infant, gasping against gravity for the first time, awakens to the music of its own existence.

The Heart's Reversal

In utero, the fetus lives in a world where oxygen is borrowed. Blood is shunted through clever detours—the foramen ovale, ductus arteriosus, and ductus venosus— allowing life to flourish without breath. But when the first inhalation draws air into the lungs, pulmonary vessels dilate in an instant. Resistance falls, and the heart, that faithful drummer, redirects its rhythm toward independence.

What was once a circuit shared with the mother becomes a self-contained universe. The placenta, which had served as heart, lung, and liver, retires in an act of divine surrender. The newborn, now the keeper of its own circulation, claims its sovereignty.

I often think of this moment as the soul's declaration of individuality—a silent, rhythmic "I am" that pulses through the tiny chest, a whisper of the infinite taking form.

The Breath of the Divine

The first cry is not just a reflex; it is a proclamation. It pierces the sterile air of the delivery room with a message older than humanity itself.

Before that cry, the lungs are oceans. They glisten with fetal fluid, their alveoli collapsed, awaiting the baptism of air. With the onset of labor and the hormonal surge of catecholamines, the fluid begins to clear. Then, when the newborn draws in the first breath, surfactant—nature's molecular lubricant—spreads across the alveolar lining, lowering surface tension, allowing the lungs to bloom like flowers opening at dawn.

For a full-term infant, this process is seamless. For the premature, it is a war. Without sufficient surfactant, each breath collapses what the last one built, like waves undoing a sandcastle. In these moments, our machines become extensions of divine mercy. We deliver pressure, oxygen, and artificial surfactant, trying to mimic the delicate physics of creation itself.

When a preemie's chest rises for the first time under our care, it feels less like a medical procedure and more like witnessing resurrection.

Of Warmth and Wonder

Inside the womb, temperature is constant, like the eternal embrace of the divine feminine. Outside, the newborn is

23

stripped bare before a world that is both wondrous and harsh. Its skin, thin as paper, releases heat faster than it can be made. The struggle to stay warm is the infant's first solitary challenge.

We swaddle them in light—radiant warmers, incubators, polyethylene wraps—re-creating the comfort of the womb. The incubator hums softly, like a metallic heart, its walls glowing with the golden hue of sunrise. Within it, the baby's temperature is monitored not as a number, but as a prayer we keep vigil over.

I have always found something profoundly symbolic in thermoregulation: the art of preserving warmth when the world is cold. It mirrors what we do as healers—maintaining the fragile flame of life against the drafts of uncertainty.

The Inner Alchemy of Independence

The moment the umbilical cord is cut, the newborn must find sustenance from within. The placenta, which once delivered glucose, amino acids, and hormones, is gone. The infant's liver, once dormant, awakens to perform its alchemy—turning stored glycogen into sugar, synthesizing energy from its own reserves.

Hormones such as cortisol and adrenaline surge, not as stress, but as initiation. The body learns self-governance. The newborn, even in its helplessness, declares autonomy at the molecular level.

In the premature infant, this declaration often falters. Hypoglycemia lurks, threatening the brain's delicate circuitry. Yet, as with every crisis in the NICU, it becomes an invitation for human hands to bridge nature's gap—a reminder that even when biology falters, compassion completes the circuit.

The Evolution of Care

In decades past, our interventions were crude yet earnest. We ventilated with force, sedated without nuance, and fed through tubes that bypassed nature's rhythms. We kept babies alive, but sometimes at the cost of their delicate unfolding.

Today, we have learned a gentler way. Neonatal care has evolved from domination to partnership.

- **Non-invasive ventilation**—CPAP, NIPPV, and high-flow cannula—supports the infant's own efforts rather than replacing them.

- **Volume-targeted ventilation** and **NAVA** align the machine's rhythm with the baby's, as though technology itself has learned to listen.

- **Less invasive surfactant therapy (LISA/MIST)** delivers the life-saving compound through a whisper-thin catheter, preserving the sanctity of spontaneous breathing.

- **AI-guided nutrition** and **personalized parenteral feeds** now mirror the wisdom of the placenta, tailoring nutrients to each infant's metabolic signature.

In these advances, I see not the triumph of science alone, but its redemption—an evolution from control to communion.

Case Vignette | Baby Hope: A 24-Week Preemie's Fight to Breathe

At twenty-four weeks' gestation, Baby Hope entered the world weighing scarcely six hundred grams—no larger than my palm, her skin translucent like rose-colored glass. Her cry, faint as a whisper, carried the defiance of a soul unwilling to yield.

She was born by emergency cesarean after her mother's body succumbed to severe preeclampsia and placental abruption. The operating room became a theatre of urgency. Under the sterile lights, time slowed as we received her fragile body—heart fluttering, lungs silent.

We moved as one organism: the respiratory therapist sealing a tiny mask over her face, the nurse adjusting the warmer, me threading the endotracheal tube as delicately as threading a prayer. Surfactant dripped into her lungs, liquid gold spreading life across collapsing alveoli.

Numbers flickered—oxygen saturation 60%, 70%, 85%— each one a rung on the ladder from uncertainty to hope.

Her isolette became her new womb, a glass sanctuary glowing with blue light and quiet vigilance. High-frequency ventilation provided hundreds of gentle puffs each minute. Intravenous lines snaked through her paper-thin skin, delivering nutrition, antibiotics, and measured hope.

Her parents stood outside, hands pressed against the incubator wall—love separated by plastic yet undiminished. A nurse tucked a small heart-shaped cloth, perfumed with her mother's scent, beside her head. Science met tenderness in that moment; both were necessary, both sacred.

Days passed like waves upon an endless shore. Day 5: pneumothorax—air trapped in her chest. A swift needle decompression freed her lungs to rise again. Day 9: patent ductus arteriosus—treated with Ibuprofen/Acetaminophen and prayer. Day 12: a small brain bleed, Grade II. Each crisis a crucible, each recovery a hymn.

Weeks became months. Gentle ventilation, caffeine for apnea, cautious oxygen titration—all tiny steps toward autonomy. On her hundredth day, we heard her first unaided cry. The sound was ragged, imperfect, glorious.

When her mother finally held her skin-to-skin, Hope's heart rate steadied, her breathing synced with the rhythm that had once nourished her in the womb. There are few miracles as quiet and complete as that—the reunion of two heartbeats once separated by necessity.

After 128 days, she left our unit on low-flow oxygen, a silver thread of air trailing her like a ribbon of triumph. She went home not merely as a survivor, but as a testament to the exquisite partnership between human skill and divine mercy.

In her, I saw reflected the purpose of our calling: to guard the threshold between heaven and earth.

Reflections | The Sacredness of Beginnings

Each birth I attend feels like standing before a burning bush—holy ground disguised as sterile tile. I approach it with awe and trembling. The science is intricate, the outcomes uncertain, yet the moment itself is eternal.

To witness the first breath is to glimpse the divine exhale that set creation into motion. To cradle a life that should not yet exist outside the womb is to hold a fragment of eternity in mortal hands.

I do not see myself merely as a physician. I am a participant in a mystery—an intermediary between biology and the ineffable. The NICU, with its wires and monitors, is a modern temple where technology bows to love, and where every breath reminds us that grace is measurable in milliliters and heartbeats.

The newborn embodies the sacred union of opposites—the divine masculine and feminine, the lover and the beloved—manifesting through flesh. In each of these fragile bodies, I see the ongoing act of creation, as if God were still speaking, "Let there be life."

To stand at that threshold is an honor beyond profession. It is a calling, a covenant, and a continual awakening to the mystery of beginnings.

Chapter 2 – When Life Hangs by a Thread

There are nights when the hospital breathes with me—when the hallways hold their air the way I do before threading a tube no wider than a coffee stirrer into a throat the size of a drinking straw. On those nights, the fluorescent lights seem kinder, and the monitors blink like votive candles in a chapel built of glass and alarms. Those are also the nights when the calendar matters more than the clock: **22 weeks, 23, 24, 25**—numbers that decide whether we are midwives to possibility or guardians of comfort.

We call it the **gray zone**: the stretch of gestation between 22 and 25 weeks where the map ends and the compass of compassion begins. I used to imagine "gray" as dull, a color without conviction. Here, it is a luminous silver—hard to grasp, shimmering with hope and doubt, alive with the stubborn defiance of a child who may never weigh a full pound. There are no straight lines in this territory, only contour lines—gestational age, estimated fetal weight, antenatal steroids received or not, a heartbeat strong or struggling, membranes ruptured for an hour or a week, parents who have named their son already or who haven't dared learn his sex. Every contour shifts the altitude of our decisions.

We teach the gray zone to our trainees as if it were a decision tree. In truth, it is a forest.

The Threshold

At **22 weeks**, medicine stands at the edge of a cliff. We can see the far shore but lack a bridge sturdy enough to guarantee the crossing. Sometimes a path appears—a larger baby than expected, a heartbeat that refuses to dim, a mother whose waters have sealed—yet so often, we face wind and rain and darkness. Comfort care is not failure here. It is fidelity: to the child's fragility, to the family's reality, to the truth that love does not always mean doing more.

At **25 weeks**, we step onto firmer ground. Our tools—ventilators, surfactant, intravenous nutrition, gentle warmth, and time—have purchase. Survival becomes a word we can say without apology, though not without caveat. The path still climbs steeply through storms of infection, bleeding, lung disease, and retinopathy—but we know the trail.

Between those edges—**23 to 24 weeks**—we ask different questions. Not "Can we?" but "Should we, and how?" Not "Will this baby live?" but "What kind of life are we inviting them toward, and are we willing to walk with this family the entire way, whatever the outcome?" This is where statistics fade to background music and **values** step to the microphone.

I have sat at hundreds of bedsides in that borderland, a chair pulled close, my hands unclenched and visible, my voice as steady as the facts will allow. Every conversation is new because every love story is new. There is no algorithm for what a parent hopes, or fears, or can endure. There is only the practice of listening deeply enough to hear the **meaning** behind the words.

The Conversation Before the Cry

We call it **antenatal counseling**, but the sterile phrase disguises what it truly is: a vigil around a possibility. We bring a paper with shaded bars—survival, survival without major impairment, the range of outcomes like a weather forecast that stops short of tomorrow. We speak in careful sentences:

"Your baby is **22 weeks and 6 days**."

"Some centers offer resuscitation at this age; some do not."

"Steroids you received will help mature the lungs and brain."

"We will honor the choice you make together."

I have learned not to rush. The parents need to hear **their own voices** deciding. I often ask, "Tell me about your baby. Do you have a name?" A name draws the future into the room. It humanizes the decision while keeping us honest about uncertainty. Sometimes they answer without breath, as if the name itself were breakable. Sometimes they cannot, and that too is holy.

In these conversations, we traffic not in guarantees but in **integrity**. I name that integrity out loud: "My commitment is to the truth as we know it, and to you as you are. We can walk a path of maximal intervention; we can walk a path of comfort. Both are paths of love."

What I do not say—but carry like a small stone in my pocket—is my own moral exposure. If they choose intensive care, I will marshal a team to fight for breath. If they choose comfort, I will show them how to hold their baby without fear. Either way, I will watch a life measure itself in minutes and miracles. And I will go home and leave the bathroom light on while I shower, grateful to share the dark with something gentle.

Ethics That Breathe

In medical school, they taught us four pillars: **autonomy, beneficence, non-maleficence, justice**. In the NICU, they do not sit like pillars; they **move** like dancers.

Autonomy: We honor the parents' right to make informed choices for their child. But autonomy is not abandonment. Consent is not a signature; it is a relationship. I have learned that autonomy grows in the soil of trust—nourished by time, watered by plain speech, sheltering under the canopy of our presence.

Beneficence: To act in the patient's best interest. Whose best interest, when the patient is a child and the consequences ripple through a family for decades? Beneficence is the promise to keep the child's good at the center, and to keep re-defining that good as the story unfolds.

Non-maleficence: Do no harm. Sometimes the harm is what we do; sometimes the harm is what we refuse to do. I have caused pain with a needle and prevented suffering with a hand left still. The question in the gray zone is seldom "harm or no harm?" but "**which harm**, toward what hope?"

Justice: Equity in access and fairness in resource. Justice is the quiet question underneath the loud ones: who gets high-tech care, who gets transferred, whose zip code writes their outcomes before I ever meet them? Justice asks me to confront the social weather systems that blow through our unit and to resist moral weather reports that turn prejudice into prophecy.

These principles are not abstractions in the gray zone; they are the **grammar** of our speech and the cadence of our care. They shape how we speak about "futility"—a word I approach like broken glass. Futility is not a judgment of a life's value; it is a limit of an **intervention's** usefulness. When I say a treatment is futile, I mean it cannot achieve the goal **we** have agreed upon—not that the patient is beyond the reach of meaning.

Consent, Shared Decision-Making, and the Ache of Conscience

Pediatrics is a triangle: child, parent, clinician. In the periviable space, the child's own voice is silent, and the triangle becomes a duet between the parents' love and our professional duty. **Parental consent** is the legal spine; **shared decision-making** is the musculature that lets us move with grace.

Some parents want us to lead—"Doctor, tell us what to do." My answer is an invitation: "Let me tell you what I can do, and what I cannot, and what it might mean. Then we'll decide **together**." Others come with strong convictions shaped by faith, culture, or prior loss. I have learned to step into those convictions with respect—never to argue with grief, never to take hope hostage with statistics. We **translate** for one another—me, converting our NICU dialect into human speech; they, translating their longing into choices we can act upon.

And then there is **moral distress**—the ache when our sense of right action collides with what we are required to do. I have felt it as a heat across the sternum when asked to escalate care in a child whose body seems to be telling us "Enough," and as a coldness in my arms when we withdraw therapies that have been our constant companions. My nurses feel it when they see suffering stretched like a taut thread across weeks; our parents feel it when love points in two directions at once.

35

We make room for that ache. We debrief. We name what is heavy. We remind each other that conscience is not a problem to solve; it is the **instrument** by which we remain human.

Gabriel's First Cry

That night, the phone rang while the unit was three beeps away from calm. "Twenty-two weeks and six days," the charge nurse said, her voice even. "Transfer from a community hospital. Membranes ruptured. Contractions every three minutes. Steroids started. Magnesium for neuroprotection. Parents want to talk."

By the time I entered the room, **Maria** lay on her side, breathing through a contraction, **Daniel** holding her shoulder like an anchor. On the bedside tray: a printout titled "Periviable Birth." I pulled a chair close.

"We are in the gray zone," I began, and watched their eyes. They were already there—wide, searching, filled with both fear and a clarity born of waiting years for this child. "Tell me about your baby," I said. "Do you have a name?"

"**Gabriel**," Maria whispered. "God's messenger."

We talked for forty minutes. I spoke plainly: survival at this age is possible but not promised; the pathway is long; the burdens are heavy. I did not shrink from the words "brain bleed," "lung disease," "infection," "long stay," but

I positioned them as terrain we might encounter—not as destiny. I told them we would honor **either** path: comfort care, wrapped in their arms, or full resuscitation with every tool we own. I named both as love.

"We want to try," Daniel said finally, the sentence landing like a blessing. "He kicks when I read to him. He's telling us to try."

"Then we will," I said, and meant **we**.

At **2:43 a.m.**, the room filled with purposeful quiet. The obstetrician delivered Gabriel by a careful, trembling cesarean: **510 grams** of luminous fragility, a body more idea than matter. For an instant, he lay still—then a **sound** escaped him, thin as a reed in the wind and yet undeniable. Not quite a cry; a **claim**.

We wrapped him in polyethylene to preserve heat, slipped the smallest endotracheal tube between vocal cords still more cartilage than music, and instilled surfactant that spread like oil upon water across alveoli begging for physics to bend in their favor. Oxygen climbed in flickers—60, 70, 85—as if the monitor itself were praying.

In the NICU, we placed him inside the isolette, that bright womb made by human hands. High-frequency ventilation offered hundreds of tiny breaths per minute, each a nudge toward life. Lines entered his body like threads of light—intravenous nutrition, antibiotics, disciplined fluids. He startled at touch, quivered at sound, yet settled when his mother's voice fluttered over him. We tucked a heart-scented cloth by his cheek, a small bridge between worlds.

I charted: *"Male infant, 22+6, 478g. Intubated in delivery room. Surfactant x1. HFOV initiated. FiO2 0.35. Mean airway pressure 12. Temperature on admission 36.5°C with polyethylene wrap. Parents counseled extensively; wish to proceed with full support."* The clinical scaffolding of a story that would, for the family, be written in a different language—of grams and days, of firsts and almosts.

Days became tide charts. **Day 5:** the right lung compressed—**pneumothorax.** I slipped a needle between ribs, felt the hiss of trapped air surrender to the room. **Day 9:** the **ductus arteriosus** refused to close and shunted blood away from promise. We gave ibuprofen, and the ductus loosened its grip. **Day 12:** ultrasound—**grade II intraventricular hemorrhage.** Not catastrophic, but a reminder that the brain, too, walks a tightrope.

At **24 weeks,** a **pulmonary hemorrhage** turned the ventilator's whisper into a wet rattle. We met in a circle—neonatology, nursing, respiratory, social work, chaplain, ethics. I have grown to love these circles. They insist we are not heroes alone but a **community** with a single patient at the center.

"Maria, Daniel," I said, careful not to crowd their grief, "Gabriel has shown us a fierce will. This bleeding adds risk. We can continue maximal support. We can also decide together to redirect toward comfort. There is no wrong choice—only the choice that matches your love."

Daniel's jaw shook. "He keeps fighting," he said. "So do we. For now, we keep going. If you tell us there's no more path, we will trust you. But for now... he's telling us to stay."

We stayed.

By **day 50**, the unit's tempo softened. The staff began to time their breaks by Gabriel's feeding schedule. I saw nurses tuck notes into his chart— "Opened his eyes with Mom's song"—and respiratory therapists bragging to one another when they weaned the oxygen by **one** percent. When Maria finally held him **skin-to-skin**, the room leaned in. The monitor found a steadier rhythm as if the numbers themselves had curled up and listened to her heart.

At **25 weeks' corrected age**, he had doubled his weight to **900 grams**. He still rode the ventilator's ghost, still needed lines, still flinched at light. But a new word entered the room: **possibility**.

I know that not every story resolves into discharge photos and cupcakes in the break room. Sometimes the story turns toward comfort, toward a small baptism of tears and silence, the holy weight of a child who teaches love in hours. I have walked that road too. The measure of a good outcome is not always longevity; it is **fidelity**—to truth, to tenderness, to the child's pace. With Gabriel, fidelity meant staying in the fight. With another baby tomorrow, fidelity might mean a blanket, a song, and a dawn where we count breaths the way pilgrims count beads.

What We Owe in the Gray

When parents ask me, "What would you do if this were your child?" I answer the only honest way I know: "I would gather the people I love, listen to the doctors I trust, and choose the path that matches our deepest values. Then I would want those doctors to **stay** with me, whichever path I chose."

That is what we owe: **presence**. It is the most underestimated therapy in the NICU formulary. Presence does not fix a hemorrhage or prevent an infection. It does something rarer: it restores **meaning** when meaning thins. It tells the parents, "You are not alone." It tells the team, "We are not instruments, we are **witnesses**." It tells the infant, in ways biology may yet measure, "You are beloved."

We also owe **clarity** without cruelty. Euphemism is a sedative with side effects. Parents deserve to know what we know, to hold it without us hiding behind jargon. They also deserve **hope** curated carefully: not counterfeit certainty, but the invitation to notice small victories—one less desaturation overnight, a gram gained, a day without a fever—as chapters in a book we are still writing.

We owe one another **rituals** of resilience. In our unit, we pause when a baby dies—alarms silenced, lights dimmed, hands on the warmer. We say the name out loud. When a baby hits a milestone, we tape a paper butterfly to the isolette. When a parent is brave—and they always are—we say so on rounds. These rituals are our counter-narratives to burnout; they are how we metabolize grief into service.

And we owe **justice** beyond our walls. The gray zone does not treat all families equally. Some travel across counties because their hospital cannot offer certain therapies. Some cannot miss work to sit at a bedside, and so their love looks like absence. I fight for transfers, for insurance approvals, for lactation supplies and transportation vouchers, because justice begins small and then grows. I cannot fix the weather, but I can open an umbrella.

A Theology of Uncertainty

People sometimes ask how I reconcile my faith with my work, as if science were a language God cannot speak. In the gray zone, uncertainty is not the enemy of faith; it is the **terrain** where faith learns to walk. Faith here does not predict; it **accompanies**. It does not guarantee outcomes; it guarantees **presence**. In this way, it looks remarkably like medicine at its best.

When I place my gloved hand on a baby's foot light as moth wing, I feel the hum of the incubator and something else—an invitation to humility. The child is both

biological and **mystical**, both alveoli and awe. Every decision I make must honor both truths. The ventilator settings are not secular; the prayers are not unscientific. They are different dialects of the same language—care.

Closing Reflections: The Thread That Holds

I used to imagine the "thread" in the phrase *when life hangs by a thread* as precarious, something that might snap at any moment. Now I see it differently. The thread is **strong**—braided from parental love, team vigilance, careful technique, ethical clarity, and the child's will. It may be thin, but it is tensile. We are weavers, not merely watchers.

Sometimes that thread carries a child across the chasm. Sometimes it lowers them gently into the arms that wait beyond sight. Either way, our hands are on it together.

Gabriel taught me again what the gray zone always teaches: that uncertainty is a place, not a punishment; that love is a decision repeated hourly; that the distance between science and sacrament is the span of a nurse's palm on a mother's back at 3 a.m.

When I left the hospital on the morning Gabriel reached 25 weeks corrected, the sky over the parking lot was pearl gray, the color of **becoming**. I breathed the cold air and whispered a benediction I have learned to offer without words: *May we be worthy of this work. May we stay human* *while we practice the impossible. May we be present until the end—whatever end arrives.*

Reflection & Practice Touchstones

1. **Language of Honesty:** What phrases help you convey risk without stealing hope? Which words land as weapons, and which as welcome?

2. **Fidelity Over Fixing:** In a recent gray-zone case, what did fidelity ask of you? Was it intervention or restraint—or both at different times?

3. **Moral Distress Hygiene:** How do you and your team discharge moral heat—huddles, debriefs, rituals? What would make those practices more regular and restorative?

4. **Justice at the Bedside:** Identify one small, actionable step to reduce inequity for a current NICU family (transportation, translation, lactation support, social work follow-through). Do it this week.

5. **Presence as Therapy:** Where did your presence—unhurried, attentive, embodied—make a difference today? Name it. Share it with a colleague.

6.   **Meaning-Making with Families:** What is one question you can add to antenatal counseling that invites values into the room? (e.g., "What would a good day look like for your baby?")

7.   **Self-Compassion:** What boundary or practice keeps your heart open without breaking? Schedule it; treat it as clinical duty.

Chapter 3 - The Biology of Grief

The Body Remembers

Grief is not merely an emotion—it is a full-body phenomenon. When loss enters a human life, it reverberates through the nervous system, the immune response, and even the molecular codes of the cells that hold memory. What begins as a spiritual and emotional ache soon becomes a physiological reality. The heart races, sleep fragments, appetite fades, and the immune system weakens. Every beat and breath becomes an echo of what the body has lost.

In perinatal loss, this process is especially profound. The attachment begins not at birth but long before it—during the months of gestation when a parent's physiology synchronizes with a growing life. Hormones of bonding, anticipation, and nurturing surge through the bloodstream. When that bond is broken, the entire system is thrown into disarray.

For healthcare providers who witness this repeatedly in the neonatal intensive care unit, the grief takes on a quieter but equally real biological form. Though less personal, the cumulative exposure to death, fragility, and family sorrow can erode emotional resilience, altering the same stress pathways that govern grief in parents. The biology of mourning, then, is a universal story—one that unites patient and provider alike through shared human vulnerability.

The Neurobiology of Grief

When loss occurs, the brain reacts as if confronted by danger. The amygdala—the sentinel of emotional alarm—fires signals that cascade through the hypothalamus, activating the body's fight-or-flight response. Cortisol and catecholamines surge into circulation, preparing the body to confront threat or flee from it. But this time, the enemy is invisible. There is no danger to escape, no wound to heal—only absence.

The amygdala heightens emotional reactivity, while the prefrontal cortex—the part responsible for judgment and regulation—loses its steady grip, leaving the bereaved in waves of uncontrollable emotion or indecision. The hippocampus, burdened by the chemical wash of stress, falters in forming new memories, explaining the disorientation and forgetfulness of early grief. Meanwhile, the nucleus accumbens—the brain's center for motivation and reward—remains tied to the image of the loved one, perpetuating yearning and the painful drive to reconnect.

In this neurochemical storm, cortisol, oxytocin, and endogenous opioids each play paradoxical roles. Cortisol prepares the body for stress but, when prolonged, damages immunity and cognitive clarity. Oxytocin—the hormone of bonding—deepens the sense of longing by keeping attachment circuits alive even in the absence of the loved one. The body continues to "wait" for return. Endogenous opioids, meant to dull pain, may numb emotional vitality when chronically elevated. Thus, the biology of grief becomes a mirror of love itself—what once bonded now binds the sufferer to their loss.

The Physiology of Sorrow

Every organ system participates in grief. The cardiovascular system bears the weight of heightened sympathetic tone—racing heart, elevated blood pressure, and, in some cases, Takotsubo cardiomyopathy, aptly named "broken heart syndrome." The endocrine system suffers from hormonal imbalance as the hypothalamic-pituitary-adrenal axis remains locked in overdrive. The immune system weakens, allowing inflammation to take root, increasing vulnerability to illness.

Fatigue, insomnia, chest tightness, headaches, and digestive troubles are common physical manifestations. They are the body's language for what the soul cannot yet articulate. In the bereaved parent, these symptoms are often amplified by the sudden hormonal withdrawal after pregnancy—the body that once sustained life must now endure its own physiological mourning.

Parental and Provider Grief: Two Faces of the Same Wound

Though the experience of loss differs between parents and healthcare providers, the body's response follows the same biological symphony of stress and sorrow.

For a parent, the loss of a child represents a primal rupture—the severing of an attachment woven into the deepest layers of identity. The brain's limbic system, wired for protection and caregiving, cannot reconcile the contradiction of life and death intertwined. The yearning to hold, nurture, and protect remains active even in absence, prolonging the physiological stress response. Such intensity of grief often leads to profound hormonal and immune dysregulation. Cortisol levels may remain high for months, sleep becomes fragmented, and the emotional brain resists the passage of time. Without support, the parent risks sliding into prolonged grief disorder, depression, or cognitive fatigue that clouds judgment and memory.

For the healthcare provider, the wound is subtler but accumulative. Exposure to repeated deaths, critical illnesses, and family distress can result in what some call **"grief stress injury."** Each loss leaves a trace within the nervous system, a micro-trauma that can compound into burnout or emotional detachment. While the attachment bond is not as intimate as that of a parent, the repetitive nature of professional loss can mirror chronic stress physiology: increased sympathetic arousal, headaches, palpitations, and insomnia.

The parent's grief burns like a sudden inferno; the provider's grief smolders quietly over years. Both are rooted in the same human circuitry of empathy and loss, and both demand acknowledgment and care.

Hormones, Stress, and the HPA Axis

At the core of grief's biology lies the hypothalamic-pituitary-adrenal (HPA) axis, a finely tuned system designed to protect against threat. Upon loss, cortisol floods the bloodstream, keeping the body alert and restless. While helpful in the short term, chronic cortisol elevation weakens immunity, disrupts metabolism, and interferes with sleep cycles. The diurnal rhythm of cortisol—the gentle rise in morning, the fall by evening—flattens, leaving the bereaved in a state of constant activation.

Catecholamines such as adrenaline and norepinephrine reinforce this cycle, maintaining high blood pressure and muscular tension. Some individuals experience shortness of breath, chest pain, or palpitations that mimic heart disease but are rooted in emotional distress.

Meanwhile, oxytocin sustains the emotional bond even in the face of loss. In prolonged grief, this hormone remains elevated, perpetuating the yearning for connection. The body clings to the relationship on a cellular level, as if refusing to accept separation.

Together, these hormonal shifts explain why grief is both exhausting and persistent. The body's alarm system, designed for short bursts of survival stress, becomes a long-term state of physiological mourning.

The Mind–Body Imprint of Perinatal Loss

Perinatal loss is unique in that it occurs at the intersection of biology and becoming. During pregnancy, hormonal and neurochemical changes prepare both parents—especially the mother—for nurturing. Oxytocin, prolactin, and endorphins orchestrate the emotional readiness for caregiving. When the expected child dies, the entire system that anticipated attachment collapses without resolution.

The psychological symptoms—nightmares, intrusive memories, guilt, and emotional numbness—are matched by somatic echoes: tightness in the chest, pain in the abdomen, insomnia, and even phantom sensations of fetal movement. Many women describe an aching "emptiness" in the womb or an invisible weight pressing upon the heart. Fathers, too, experience physical restlessness, muscle tension, and chronic fatigue as the body processes an unspeakable loss through movement and sleepless nights.

This intertwining of mind and body forms what trauma theorists call **embodied grief**. The nervous system does not easily distinguish emotional pain from physical threat. It keeps the body in a state of readiness long after the loss, awaiting a reunion that never comes.

Resilience and Post-Traumatic Growth

Grief need not end in pathology. Within its depths lies the potential for transformation. **Resilience** is the capacity to maintain stable function despite trauma, while **post-traumatic growth (PTG)** represents the evolution of a new identity shaped by suffering.

Resilient individuals often display adaptive regulation of their stress systems—their cortisol rhythms recover faster, and their autonomic balance returns more readily to baseline. But growth requires struggle. PTG often emerges after a prolonged period of cognitive dissonance when one's fundamental beliefs about life and fairness are shattered and slowly rebuilt.

The key mechanism for such transformation is **meaning-making**—the active re-construction of one's worldview to accommodate the loss. Positive coping strategies such as journaling, therapy, mindfulness, prayer, and compassionate conversation strengthen neuroplasticity and re-establish prefrontal control over the amygdala's distress signals.

Biologically, genes such as *FKBP5* and *CRHR1*—which regulate stress reactivity—may modulate vulnerability or resilience to grief. Epigenetic studies suggest that even trauma-induced changes in these genes can be reversed through sustained healing environments. Neurochemicals like **neuropeptide Y (NPY)** and **brain-derived neurotrophic factor (BDNF)** further enhance the brain's capacity to adapt, underscoring that recovery from grief is not only psychological but molecular.

The Healing Power of Connection

If grief is a biological disconnection, healing begins with reconnection. Human touch, empathy, and shared mourning can regulate the very systems that loss destabilizes. When a grieving person is held, listened to, or comforted, oxytocin rises and cortisol falls. The parasympathetic nervous system—the body's calming branch—awakens.

Social support acts as both buffer and balm. Studies consistently show that individuals with strong social networks recover more rapidly from bereavement. In the context of perinatal loss, this includes family-centered care, support groups, remembrance rituals, and open acknowledgment of both parents' grief.

Fathers, however, often stand outside this circle of care. Cultural expectations of stoicism leave them unseen. Their biology, too, suffers silently—the suppressed emotions manifesting as hypertension, insomnia, or depression. Yet when men are invited into the grieving process—when they are encouraged to speak, cry, and remember—their physiological stress markers improve. Their stories, like those of mothers, need space to breathe.

It is within this landscape of silent suffering that the following vignette unfolds—one that captures the quiet anguish of paternal grief and the profound truth that love, even in silence, leaves a biological echo.

Case Vignette: "Silent Monitors — A Father's Unspoken Pain"

The delivery room was unusually quiet. The rhythmic beeping of the fetal monitor—a sound that once symbolized reassurance—had gone still. The silence that followed was deafening. **Stella** lay on the bed, pale and tear-streaked, while **Dr. Tajon** gently explained that despite all efforts, the baby's heart had stopped just hours before delivery.

Standing in the corner, **Jofe,** her husband, watched everything unfold. He had spent the last three nights pacing hospital corridors, praying for a miracle. At thirty-six weeks, their daughter was supposed to be safe. He had assembled the crib just a week before, tightening each screw with the excitement of a first-time father. Now, his hands hung uselessly at his sides, trembling.

When the nurse asked if he wanted to hold his daughter, he hesitated. His wife nodded, so he did. Wrapped in a white blanket, her still body rested lightly in his arms. Her tiny fingers curled against his palm—perfect, delicate, and heartbreakingly still. He tried to speak but no words came out. His tears fell silently, leaving small, wet circles on her blanket.

Later, as Stella was wheeled to postpartum recovery, Jofe stayed behind to sign paperwork. **"Disposition of remains,"** the form said. He stared at those words for a long time, unable to comprehend how fatherhood could begin and end with a signature.

Over the next few days, Stella was surrounded by friends, family, and nurses offering comfort. Flowers arrived, condolences were sent, and a social worker visited daily. But no one asked Jofe how he was doing. He became the silent caretaker—holding his wife when she sobbed, organizing funeral details, returning baby gifts. At night, he sat in the dark nursery, the soft glow of the baby monitor casting light on an empty crib.

His grief had no outlet. Society had taught him to be the strong one—the protector, the provider. When he tried to speak about the loss at work, his colleagues awkwardly changed the subject or said, "At least she's young—you can try again."

Weeks turned to months. Stella joined a perinatal loss support group, where she found solace in sharing her story. Jofe went once but didn't return. "It's not for me," he said. Instead, he began running before dawn—mile after mile, pounding the pavement, chasing the silence that now filled their home.

One night, Stella found him sitting in the nursery again, staring at the monitor. "I keep hearing her," he whispered. "That soft static... it's like she's still here." Tears welled in his eyes for the first time in months. Stella knelt beside him, and for the first time, they grieved together.

Discussion and Reflection

"Silent Monitors" illuminates an often-overlooked dimension of perinatal loss—the father's unspoken grief. While mothers receive medical and emotional care, fathers frequently assume the role of silent witnesses, suppressing their pain beneath the weight of duty.

This story reflects several critical truths.

First, **men's grief is often invisible.** Social norms discourage vulnerability, and healthcare systems rarely direct bereavement resources toward fathers.

Second, **gendered expectations distort healing.** Men who are taught to be stoic may internalize sorrow, leading to physiological manifestations—hypertension, sleep disturbance, or depression.

Finally, **inclusion is healing.** When fathers are invited into bereavement rituals, counseling, or remembrance practices, their emotional expression becomes part of a shared recovery that strengthens the entire family system.

In the quiet hum of the "silent monitors," Jofe's pain becomes the echo of countless fathers who grieve in shadows. His story reminds clinicians that every loss resonates beyond the mother's body—it reverberates through both hearts that dreamed of life. Healing begins not in silence, but in the sacred act of being heard.

PART II

The Human
Heart of Healing

"Grief is love that has nowhere to go, until we give it form through remembrance." Arwin M. Valencia, MD

Chapter 4 – The Parents' Journey

Grief in the neonatal and perinatal setting is unlike any other human experience. It occurs at the intersection of hope and heartbreak—where dreams once measured in heartbeats are silenced before they can take root in the world. Parents who lose a child during pregnancy, birth, or shortly thereafter face a unique and profound kind of mourning: they grieve not only a life but a lifetime of imagined moments that will never unfold. The nursery that was meant to cradle new beginnings becomes a sacred space of remembrance. In this quiet void, healing is not about moving on but about learning to live with a love that no longer has a physical form.

The Phases of a Parent's Grief

Although grief has been mapped through psychological models such as the Kübler-Ross stages—shock, denial, anger, bargaining, depression, and acceptance—real-life grief defies linearity. Parents do not move through these emotions in predictable order; they oscillate, regress, leap forward, and fall back, as if caught between two tides— one of love, the other of loss.

Shock and Denial often arrive as protective veils. The brain, overwhelmed by unbearable reality, dulls perception so the heart can survive. A mother may awaken from anesthesia and ask, "When can I hold my baby?"

before the room's silence gives her the answer. A father may pace the hospital hallway, believing any moment will bring the sound of his child's cry. Denial, in these moments, is not ignorance—it is mercy.

As reality settles, **guilt** begins to whisper. Parents replay every moment of pregnancy or delivery, searching for what they could have done differently. Mothers wonder if an extra hour of rest, a different doctor, a stricter diet might have changed the outcome. Fathers, too, often bear invisible guilt for not protecting their partner or child from harm. In truth, such guilt is the mind's attempt to reclaim control in a situation where there was none.

Anger may follow, raw and consuming. It can be directed at fate, medicine, God, or oneself. Sometimes it is expressed outwardly, other times buried beneath polite composure. Beneath the anger lies pain—an expression of love seeking justice for what feels unjust.

In time, **depression** settles in, not as weakness but as a natural descent into the depths of sorrow. The world appears muted. Joy feels like betrayal. Parents often describe this phase as living in grayscale, moving through routines without meaning. Healing, at this point, seems impossible—but even this stillness serves a purpose. It is the body's way of conserving energy while the spirit slowly reorganizes itself around a new reality.

Finally, **acceptance** emerges—not as relief, but as surrender. It is not forgetting the child or ceasing to love them, but learning to hold their memory in peace rather than pain. Acceptance is the quiet recognition that grief will forever be part of one's identity, like a scar that no longer bleeds but remains sensitive to touch.

These phases are not milestones to be completed but waves to be navigated. Each family's journey through them is as unique as their child's heartbeat once was.

The Inner Landscape of Parental Grief

In the clinical setting, physicians and nurses witness this landscape daily: the trembling hands that cradle a lifeless infant, the mother's empty gaze, the father's silent tears. Yet, beneath each expression of sorrow lies a universal truth—grief is love without a destination.

Grieving parents inhabit two worlds simultaneously. In one, they function as members of society, returning to work, paying bills, smiling when required. In the other, they live in sacred time, where their child is ever-present— felt in the wind, seen in dreams, remembered in every sunset. To the outside world, it may appear they are "moving on." Internally, they are learning to walk between worlds, carrying their child within them like a hidden flame.

This paradox—love enduring beyond form—demands both emotional courage and spiritual reckoning. Healing begins not when pain ends, but when meaning is rediscovered.

Communication and Compassion in the Healing Space

For healthcare providers, few tasks are as emotionally charged as delivering devastating news. The conversation that follows—the moment a parent learns that their baby's life cannot be sustained—is an encounter that shapes every memory thereafter. Words matter, but tone and presence matter more.

In the medical literature, structured frameworks like **SPIKES** (Setting, Perception, Invitation, Knowledge, Empathy, and Summarize/Strategize). and **NURSE** (Name, Understand, Respect, Support, and Explore) have been developed to guide clinicians through these encounters. Yet beyond the acronyms lies a deeper truth: compassion cannot be scripted. It must be embodied.

Breaking bad news requires courage, humility, and grace. It begins with creating safety—a quiet room, eye-level seating, time unhurried by the clock. The clinician must first *set up* the space not only physically but emotionally, grounding themselves before entering the family's storm. They must *assess perception*, gently exploring what the family already understands, for this determines how truth can be received.

When *delivering knowledge*, the most powerful words are those spoken with clarity and sincerity, free of jargon and defensiveness. A "warning shot" like "I'm afraid I have difficult news" prepares the heart for impact. What follows must be slow, deliberate, and human. Medical data offers understanding; empathy offers survival.

The *empathy* phase—the heart of this exchange—is where the NURSE principles take life. The clinician names the emotion they perceive ("I can see how painful this is"), validates it ("Anyone in your position would feel the same"), and expresses unwavering respect for the parent's strength. They offer support, not through promises of outcomes, but through presence: "You're not alone in this. We will walk through it together."

Finally, *summarizing and strategizing* gives the family something to hold onto—a sense of orientation in the chaos. Whether that means outlining comfort care options, memorial rituals, or psychological support, the act of planning restores agency to those who have just lost control over the most precious thing in their lives.

Holding Space: The Silent Ministry of Presence

Beyond words, the most profound act of care is the willingness to **hold space**. To hold space means to enter another's pain without flinching, to be still in their suffering without needing to fix it. It is an art of restraint—

offering your full presence without inserting your own discomfort or agenda.

Holding space involves radical acceptance: allowing the grieving parent to feel *everything*—the rage, the guilt, the despair—without correction or spiritual bypassing. Statements like "At least you can try again" or "Everything happens for a reason" may come from good intentions but often deepen isolation. The bereaved do not seek explanations; they seek acknowledgment.

Presence is the living expression of empathy. It is more than proximity—it is attunement. The caregiver who leans in, who maintains gentle eye contact, who allows silence to stretch without rushing to fill it, communicates a truth that words cannot: *You matter. Your pain matters. Your child matters.*

In these moments, time slows. The sterile room becomes sacred ground. The clinician and parent meet not as doctor and patient, but as two souls confronting the mystery of life and death together. This is the essence of **compassion beyond words**—the healing that arises simply from being seen, held, and accompanied through darkness.

The Empty Crib — A Mother's Testimony of Love That Transcends Time

The nursery stood ready—walls painted the soft blush of dawn, a white crib draped in lace, and a mobile of stars gently swaying in the quiet air. It was a space made sacred by anticipation. Every folded onesie, every bottle arranged with care spoke of a love already overflowing, waiting only for the moment it could finally be cradled in arms. But love, in its most mysterious expression, sometimes reveals itself not through what remains, but through what is taken away.

When I met **Donna**, she sat beside that same crib—empty, yet impossibly full. Her baby, **Tammy**, had lived for only three days. Three days of fragile breaths, whispered prayers, and the steady rhythm of machines fighting to sustain life on the thinnest thread of hope. For most, it would have seemed unbearably brief. But for Donna, it was eternity compressed into a handful of heartbeats.

The First Cry That Never Came

Donna's pregnancy had been radiant with joy. Every ultrasound felt like a benediction—the flicker of a heartbeat, the curl of a tiny hand. At 32 weeks, however, silence replaced melody. The Doppler found no rhythm, only uncertainty. "We need to deliver now," the obstetrician said softly.

Tammy entered the world in a blur of urgency. The NICU team worked in orchestrated grace—compressions, breaths, tubes, prayers. Then, a sound—a faint cry, the most fragile declaration of life. Hope surged. For three days, Donna lived in suspended time, watching the monitors dance like constellations. Each breath Tammy took was a miracle written in seconds.

But on the third night, her tiny heart began to tire. Machines fell quiet. The physician, voice trembling, whispered, "You can hold her now." No tubes, no wires—only skin to skin, heart to heart. The warmth faded, but peace arrived. "She was never mine to keep," Donna said later. "But I will forever be hers."

The Empty Crib as Altar

Friends suggested she clear the nursery—it might help her heal. But Donna couldn't. Instead, she transformed it. The crib became an altar of remembrance: a folded blanket, a candle lit each dusk, a photograph framed by love. "I used to rock her here in my dreams," she said. "Now, I come to feel her in the silence."

Preserving the nursery was not denial. It was devotion. The empty crib became a symbol of transcendence—the proof that love, once awakened, does not end. It only changes form.

The Biology of a Mother's Grief

Science confirms what Donna instinctively knew. The maternal brain is rewired during pregnancy; oxytocin and dopamine pathways carve deep emotional bonds that persist beyond the body. When loss occurs, the same regions that light up in love also activate in pain. Her milk came in though her arms were empty; her body still prepared to nurture. "My body didn't know she was gone," she whispered. "It still reached for her."

Grief, then, is not just psychological—it is biological. The body mourns with the soul. Healing requires time for both systems to realign, for neural pathways to integrate the reality of loss without erasing the love that birthed them.

The Spiritual Continuum of Love

As weeks passed, Donna began to dream. Tammy appeared not as an infant but as light—radiant, mischievous, just beyond touch. "She told me she came not to stay, but to remind me love is eternal." Grief had become her teacher, unveiling what mystics have always known: love is energy, and energy cannot be destroyed.

Donna began writing letters to her daughter. "I still sing your lullaby," one read. "Maybe that's how the angels find you." These rituals transformed sorrow into communion. They bridged two worlds—the living and the unseen.

Legacy of Light

Years later, Donna returned to the NICU—not as a patient, but as a volunteer. She sat with mothers who held their dying infants, offering silent companionship. She did not quote scripture or science. She simply whispered, "You will carry them differently, but you will carry them always."

Through her, Tammy's short life multiplied into countless acts of healing. The empty crib had given birth again—this time, to compassion.

Reflections from the Crib

When asked what healing meant to her, Donna rested her hand on the crib's edge and smiled faintly.

"People think healing means forgetting," she said. "But healing is remembering differently. The crib isn't empty anymore—it's full of every lullaby, every tear, every dream. Love didn't end when her heartbeat stopped. It became timeless."

Closing Reflection

In medicine, success is often measured by survival rates and discharge summaries. But in rooms like Donna's, where an empty crib stands both as memorial and miracle, success must be measured by something deeper—the capacity of love to transcend loss.

For every parent who leaves the hospital with empty arms, there remains a sacred truth: grief is not the absence of love but its deepest proof.

In every NICU, where science meets soul, there are unseen cribs—altars of love, repositories of tears, sanctuaries of remembrance. Within them, the light of eternal love flickers gently, reminding us that healing is not about closure—it is about continuation.

A parent's journey does not end with loss. It continues, transformed, forever echoing in the rhythm of a love that time can never silence.

Chapter 5 – The Clinician's Crossroads

There is a quiet threshold every clinician crosses at the beginning of a shift—the moment the badge clicks, the scrub top is adjusted, the familiar antiseptic scent of the hospital wraps itself around the body like a ritual garment. On one side of that threshold is ordinary life: coffee in a kitchen, laughter in a hallway, a child's drawing pinned by magnets to a refrigerator. On the other side is the intensive care unit, where life hovers close to its origins and endings, where breath is measured in fractions, where sleep and appetite and circadian rhythms submit to the unblinking cadence of monitors. The NICU is not only a place of machines and medicine; it is a school for the human heart.

Every clinician who lives here long enough comes to understand the paradox at the center of the work: the same tender empathy that allows us to respond exquisitely to suffering can, without careful tending, erode our capacity to remain present. The same connection that fuels us can deplete us. And yet, the same compassion that sometimes drains us is also the well from which meaning, resilience, and quiet joy continue to flow. This is the crossroads—**the enduring tension between compassion fatigue and compassion satisfaction**—and navigating it is as much an inner art as it is a professional skill.

The Cost and the Gift

Compassion fatigue is often called the "cost of caring," but that phrase feels too small for the weight it carries. It is not simply a late-night weariness or a passing grey mood after a hard case. It is an exhaustion that enters the body and hides in the muscles of the face, in the space behind the eyes, in the narrow place between one's breath and one's thoughts. It gathers slowly, granular as sand, grain by grain: yet another family meeting; one more resuscitation at the edge of viability; the yoke of documentation that must make poetry out of pain in the tidy syntax of the electronic record. Eventually, the grains form a shore where waves of sadness break without rest.

Clinicians experiencing this state describe irritability that surprises them, a thinning patience with colleagues or loved ones, dreams that replay the ventilator's metronome or a code called in the night. They speak of feeling less porous to joy, less moved by things that once delighted them. Some pull away; others lean in with even fiercer effort, as if speed and perfection could outrun sorrow. The mind asks dangerous questions: *Did I miss something? Was there one more thing I could have done?* These questions can be wise—they press us toward mastery—but when they become incessant, they erode the ground beneath our feet.

And yet, in the same landscape where fatigue grows, something luminous can also take root. **Compassion satisfaction** is the quiet fulfillment that arises when our work aligns with our deepest values: when a frightened parent exhales because we sat, unhurried, at eye level and spoke with honesty; when a tiny hand curls reflexively around our gloved finger; when an end-of-life vigil is held with reverence and a family leaves saying, *"You didn't just care for our baby—you cared for us."* These moments do not erase suffering, but they baptize it with meaning. They are the heart's wages, paid not in currency but in coherence: *I am doing what I am here to do.*

The clinician's task, then, is not to banish stress nor to perform invulnerability. The task is to cultivate the conditions in which satisfaction grows more quickly than fatigue—where the inner economy of the heart remains solvent, able to spend empathy without going bankrupt.

The Brain That Feels and Knows

The science of empathy helps to illuminate why this work can be both nourishing and depleting. Human brains are exquisitely designed to resonate with one another. There is, within us, a mirroring capacity that allows a clinician to "feel with" a patient—not conceptually, but viscerally. The sight of a grimace, the cadence of a cry, the posture of a body in pain—all of these activate neural networks that, in another context, would respond to our own discomfort. This is the holy circuitry that makes us human; it is also the conduit through which distress can flood the caregiver.

But empathy is not only resonance. It is also understanding. Alongside the brain's feeling centers lies a complementary system for perspective-taking—a capacity to step back, to imagine the other's interior world, to see from their vantage without losing our own. When these systems work together, clinicians can stand at the bedside with both tenderness and clarity. The resonance says, *This hurts.* The perspective says, *and this is what we must do.* Without the resonance, care becomes mechanical. Without the perspective, we drown.

From this vantage, **professional boundaries** are not cold defenses; they are a form of cognitive compassion. The mind learns to name what belongs to whom: *This anguish I sense is theirs; my role is to accompany it, not to internalize it.* The body learns signals that say it is time to pause, to breathe, to feel one's feet in the shoes that have walked so many hallways. The clinician who attends to this differentiation does not love less. They simply love sustainably.

Neuroscience gives further depth to what experience already teaches. Prolonged stress alters hormonal currents; it can erode the hippocampus's gentle work of integrating memory and shrink the prefrontal regions that make discernment possible. In other words, unmitigated exposure to suffering does not only hurt the heart; it can distort the very faculties that make careful medicine possible. The reverse is also true: practices that strengthen emotional regulation—simple breathwork before a family meeting, a micro-pause at the isolette to soften the brow and widen the attention, a colleague's hand on a shoulder after a code—help restore the brain's capacity to choose, rather than react. These are not luxuries. They are clinical tools.

The Spiritual Grammar of Care

In this place where science beats like a steady drum, another rhythm sounds—the rhythm of meaning. Many clinicians, whether religious or not, speak of moments in the unit that feel like sacrament: the hush that falls when a family sings to their dying child; the inexplicable peace that sometimes descends after chaos; the sudden alignment in a team meeting when truth is spoken without adornment and everyone in the room knows the right next thing to do. These are not mystical add-ons; they are the lifeblood of work that would otherwise be unbearable.

To see medicine as **ministry** is not to replace knowledge with faith, but to understand knowledge as a way of serving the human spirit. It is to reframe tasks—placing a line, adjusting ventilator settings, charting carefully—not as a series of technical acts but as gestures within a larger liturgy of care. The patient is never only a case; the family is never only a family; the colleague is never only a role. Each is a person, bright with worth, carrying their own histories and hopes into the room.

This lens does not immunize us against burnout. But it **re-enchants** the ordinary. When a clinician remembers that presence itself heals, the smallest acts regain their glow: the chair pulled close to the family instead of standing at the door; the honest sentence, *"I don't know, but I will find out;"* the gentle phrase spoken to an infant before an invasive procedure, *"Little one, I'm here; this will be quick."* These micro-moments revive compassion satisfaction not by adding more to do, but by seeing what we already do as meaningful.

Practices That Keep Us

A healthy professional life is braided from many strands. There is the inner practice—attention to breath, tending to the body, a brief notebook where one writes down a single moment of grace from the shift. There is the relational practice—debriefs after hard cases, peer check-ins that refuse to be performative, mentoring that acknowledges the invisible curriculum of emotional literacy. And there is the organizational practice—leaders who protect breaks and model boundaries, staffing patterns that honor human limits, rituals of remembrance for babies whose names would otherwise be lost to the sterile archive.

It helps to gather language that becomes a kind of internal oath.

I will not confuse urgency with importance.

I will not confuse capacity with calling; I cannot do all things.

I will let the team carry what I cannot, and I will carry what is mine with care.

These phrases become anchors when storms rise.

None of this negates metrics or hard outcomes; it grounds them. A unit that attends to the inner life of its clinicians does not become less excellent; it becomes more so. Fewer errors occur when attention is not brittle. Communication improves when shame is not the dominant teacher. Families feel safer when the adults in the room feel held. Babies benefit when the hands that touch them are steady not only from training, but from a heart at rest in its purpose.

A Story at the Crossroads

Case Vignette: "Dr. Salud's Dilemma"—When Doing Everything Isn't Enough

There are nights when the unit's hum sharpens into a single tone, as if the building is a tuning fork and reality has struck it. That night began with a call to the operating room: an emergency delivery at twenty-three weeks. The mother—**Lynette** -was exhausted, blood pressure rising like a tide that would not recede. The baby's tracing wavered in a language all of us could read and none of us wanted to translate.

Dr. Salud—calm, practiced, alert—stood at the warmer while the team prepared the tools that have become extensions of our bodies: 2.5 tubes lined like calligraphy, a laryngoscope gleaming under white light, plastic wrap ready to guard against the merciless dissipations of air. When the obstetrician said, "We're delivering now," the room inhaled.

The infant emerged translucent and still. Thirty seconds can be an eternity. Then a gasp—almost theoretical in its smallness—arrived, and with it the choreography: position, suction, pressure, breath. Numbers rose like faithful birds: heart rate above one hundred, color returning, air entry whistling. The baby would be named **Lyndon** later, but in those first minutes, names belong to parents and God; our work is simply to open the way.

The NICU received him as we receive all who arrive on the ledge between worlds. Oscillation lit the ventilator; surfactant slid where it needed to go. Lines were placed with the kind of attention that can feel like prayer. Lynette came to the bedside each day, pressing her hands against the isolette wall, a mother's body still telling its own story of rupture and repair. Her husband's eyes tried to become a harbor, though he too was ship and sea.

The first days were a triumph of technique. And then the cracks began to insist on being seen. Ventilator pressures crept higher; oxygen needs disobeyed; x-rays became pale clouds. Blood gases told a tale of confusion. An ultrasound spoke the sentence none of us wanted to hear: **Grade IV intraventricular hemorrhage with midline shift**—catastrophic, irreversible. The room where we read these images always feels colder after such a finding, as if the air itself recoils.

Back in the workroom, someone whispered the simplest truth: "We've done everything."

"Yes," said Dr. Salud, "and sometimes everything is still not enough."

There is a door every clinician must knock on at such times—the door that leads to a conversation where medicine and morality share the same chair. The next morning, in the conference room adjacent to the unit, beneath fluorescent lights that never learned how to be gentle, Dr. Salud sat with Lynette and her husband. He began with what he always begins with: **their** understanding. They spoke of hope and fight and the kindly nurse who had said his heart was strong. He nodded, let the words sit with dignity, then offered his own: the brain's bleeding, the lungs' struggle, the reality that machines can create a quiet that is not comfort.

"I need to ask you something very difficult," he said. "We have reached the limits of what medicine can do *for* Lyndon. Continuing may only cause him more pain. We can keep him comfortable and in your arms and let him go peacefully. Or we can continue to support him medically, knowing it will not change the outcome."

Such sentences are made of glass and mercy. They must be carried slowly.

"Are you saying there's no hope?" Lynette asked.

"There is always hope," he replied. "But sometimes hope changes its form. It becomes about peace, not prolongation."

That night, Lynette sat for hours by the isolette, tracing circles on the plexiglass with a fingertip the way a mother traces hope. She threaded her finger through the port. Lyndon's hand—no bigger than a walnut shell—curled around it. In that reflex was a sacrament: hello and goodbye braided together.

When she finally said, "We're ready," the unit shifted into the mode that only love can teach. The ventilator exhaled one last time. Lyndon was placed skin-to-skin on his mother's chest. His heart slowed, then slowed again, then found its rest. What remained was grief shaped like a mother's cry, and a stillness that felt like a shoreline after storm.

In the days that followed, Dr. Salud did what clinicians do: he rounded, he checked orders, he taught residents with gentleness, he signed and countersigned the infinite forms that codify chaos. But something in him had rearranged itself. Every alarm was a memory. Every hand he held contained the ghost of another. He read, late at night in his kitchen, the card Lynette and her husband had left:

Thank you for helping our baby live, and thank you for helping him die gently.

We know you tried everything. But what we remember most is that you stayed.

He placed the note into the notebook he carries between hospitals—a private reliquary whose pages hold small relics of humanity. Weeks later, Lynette returned with a framed photo of Lyndon resting peaceful and swaddled in her arms. She hugged him without words. "You helped us see that love doesn't end," she said. The photo found a place on his desk beside a stethoscope worn smooth by years. Some instruments pick up timbre through use.

The case did not make him harder; it made him clearer. He began to teach differently, adding to the catechism of physiology a new curriculum: that mastery includes **emotional literacy**, that the question is never only *Can we do this?* but also *Should we?* He taught that "doing everything" sometimes means stopping in time. He spoke of moral distress not as personal weakness but as the conscience's flint, striking sparks until the team gathers around what truly matters.

The Inner Oath of the Healer

When clinicians reach this crossroads—when doing more risks becoming harm and doing less risks becoming abandonment—they need more than protocols. They need an inner oath. It does not replace the Hippocratic promises; it undergirds them.

I will meet each family where they are, not where I wish them to be.

I will tell the truth gently and completely, remembering that information without presence is cruelty.

I will let science be my map and love be my compass.

I will practice boundaries as acts of care—for them and for me.

I will not mistake my exhaustion for my identity.

I will receive the balm of my colleagues' support without apology.

I will forgive myself the limitations of my humanity, for it is my humanity that makes healing possible.

These vows are not theoretical. They appear in the ordinary fabric of a shift: a physician who pauses to breathe before entering the room where a family waits; a nurse who asks a colleague to sit with her for five minutes after withdrawing support; a respiratory therapist who speaks to the baby while adjusting the ventilator, restoring language to a body surrounded by machines. They appear in the unit's culture: protected debriefs that are not optional; leaders who reward candor; schedules that leave room for sleep; ceremonies at year's end that speak the names of the children we could not keep.

The Ecosystem of a Compassionate Unit

Professional quality of life is personal and communal. A clinician can meditate and hydrate and journal until their notebooks form a stack taller than the med-surg cart, and still burn out in a system that ignores human limits. Conversely, an enlightened policy cannot save a heart that has decided it must earn its worth through endless self-expenditure. The unit becomes a living organism when policies and persons align around the same truth: we are here to care, and that includes caring for the carers.

This means staffing driven by acuity rather than inertia. It means mentorship that speaks frankly about grief and pride and the long arc of a life in medicine. It means naming the invisible labor carried by nurses who sit at bedsides through the night, by trainees who pour themselves into cases that will be footnotes in their evaluations, by attendings who hold liability and leadership in the same already-full hands. It means celebrating wins without triumphalism and narrating losses without shame.

When such an ecosystem takes shape, compassion satisfaction flourishes. People linger after shift change because they want to, not because charting trapped them. Laughter returns, properly irreverent and never cruel. The unit's reputation changes—not only for outcomes, but for presence. Families sense it without being told this is a place where medicine is practiced as an art of relationship.

The Long Obedience of Hope

What sustains a clinician across decades is not the memory of a single miraculous save, nor the mythology of heroism that medicine sometimes applies like a gold leaf over exhaustion. It is the long obedience to small fidelities. It is the knowledge that, shift after shift, we showed up. We told the truth. We touched the tiny hand, we honored the limits, we learned each time how to begin again.

There is a story in every practitioner's life that becomes an emblem. For Dr. Salud, it is Lyndon's gentle release—a night when doing less was an act of fierce care. For another, it might be a near-impossible extubation or the moment a mother laughed for the first time in weeks at her child's hiccup. For you, it will be something else altogether. These stories are not trophies; they are cairns along a long trail, stacked stones that say to those behind us: *This way. Keep going. There is meaning here.*

Closing Reflection: The Hands That Stay

In the end, the clinician's crossroads is not a single intersection we pass once. It is a place we will visit many times—on the third day of a long week, at two in the morning, halfway through a family conference when the truth is most fragile, at the white board when the numbers don't say what the heart hopes. Each time, the choice is the same: to protect the flame of our humanity while we shelter the flame of another's life.

When doing everything isn't enough, what remains is the most ancient medicine: presence that does not flee; tenderness that does not humiliate; courage that tells the truth; wisdom that knows when to hold on and when to let go. The machines will hum, the air will be dry and cool, the notes will require exactness, the protocols will ask to be followed. But beneath all that, there will be the unbroken thread of **ministry**—the sense that our hands have been entrusted with something infinitely precious.

And so, we keep an inner vigil. We place our palms on the isolette and feel, for a breath, the stillness of our own pulse. We listen for the quiet voice that once said to Dr. Salud and will say to us again: *You did not fail; you were faithful.* We pick up the stethoscope, its metal warmed by use, and step once more across the threshold, carrying with us the strange, sustaining knowledge that love, given wisely, is inexhaustible.

May our science be exacting, our boundaries kind, our presence steady.

May our labor bear fruit in the lives we touch and in the life we live.

And when we reach our own crossroad, may we choose again the path of being, the path where healing and humility walk side by side.

Chapter 6 – The Sacred Hour: End-of-Life in the NICU

There is an hour in every neonatal intensive care unit when everything seems to gather itself—lights quiet, alarms softened, footsteps instinctively slower—as though the hospital recognizes that love requires a different acoustics. Nurses sometimes call it the sacred hour. Not because of any religious rite, but because of a shared, reverent awareness: a child's life is completing itself, and we are invited to keep vigil. In that hour, medicine changes its posture. It does not turn away from knowledge or abandon skill; rather, it bends both toward a single aim—comfort. The work is no longer to reverse physiology but to companion it, to honor the body's wisdom as it lets go, and to hold a family in a circle of gentleness where goodbye can be spoken without hurry and without fear.

A Body's Farewell: The Physiology of Dying in Neonates

The physiology of dying has its own choreography—subtle, patient, at times disarmingly quiet. When life-sustaining treatments are withdrawn or when an infant's underlying condition progresses despite maximal support, the body begins a measured retreat from its most energy-intensive tasks. Breathing becomes the most visible frontier. Patterns grow irregular; a rapid cascade of small breaths can give way to long pauses, then shallow efforts that barely lift the chest. Secretions, no longer swept by strong coughs or vigorous swallows, pool in the nasopharynx and airway, creating sounds that can frighten families unfamiliar with their meaning. We name it compassionately and honestly: this noise is not suffering— it is fluid the body no longer clears. Repositioning, moisture, gentle suctioning, and calm voices do more than technology can.

Circulation follows its own slow tide. Perfusion pulls back from the skin to protect the most vital organs; hands and feet cool, color shifts to pale or blue, then to the mottled map clinicians know well. Parents often notice before we do: "His feet feel cold." We answer with truth and tenderness: "His blood is staying near his heart and brain. We'll keep him warm against you." Lethargy increases: long, drowsy stretches replace alert periods. Suck and swallow fade. The appetite that once seemed like a verdict—*she is getting stronger*—becomes irrelevant, not by neglect but by nature. Hunger belongs to bodies intent on growth; dying bodies seek rest.

Muscles soften. The little sphincters that kept order in diapers relax and release. It helps to name these things ahead of time, not as clinical data points but as signposts parents can recognize: *If this happens, it is the body's way of finishing its work. We will keep her clean, warm, and comfortable. None of this will surprise us, and none of it will change our devotion.* In the NICU, where numbers and images often govern our understanding, end-of-life physiology asks us to return to observation as a human art: skin tone under lamplight, breath against the back of a parent's hand, the unique cadence of a baby's most ordinary sighs.

Reorienting the Mission: Comfort Care as the Medicine of Presence

Comfort care in the NICU is not the absence of treatment; it is the presence of the right treatment. The orientation shifts from longevity to dignity, from aggressive correction to gentle relief, from escalation to ease. That reorientation is both ethical and practical. It is ethical because our intent is symptom relief—never hastening death, always reducing suffering. It is practical because bodies near death are exquisitely sensitive: noise becomes intrusion, light becomes glare, repeated measurements become burdens that outgrow their usefulness. The sacred hour invites us to edit the plan until only what matters remains.

We begin by transforming the environment. Lights are dimmed not to create theater but to ease overstimulated retinas; monitors are silenced when possible, and non-essential alarms are routed to the hallway so that numbers do not narrate the last moments. Warmth is provided by skin and swaddle instead of sterile heat. If ever a room should be arranged like a sanctuary, it is now. Chairs draw near and sit level with the parent's body; cords are laid aside like vines gently parted; doors are closed with the soft decisiveness of love guarding a threshold.

We widen the circle of care to include tender rituals. We encourage bathing when it is wanted, naming it as comfort and as memory, not as a clinical procedure. We offer clothing chosen by the family, not merely hospital linens, because fabric on skin can become part of a story that will be told for years. We ask about music, language, prayer—if any—and we learn a word or two in the family's mother tongue because sometimes the most merciful sentence is simply, *I am here*, spoken in the sound of home.

Skin-to-skin contact, kangaroo care, becomes not only possible but central. When a mother or father holds their child against the heart, temperature regulation stabilizes, distress decreases, and the natural hormones of attachment—oxytocin, serotonin, endorphins—do work no pharmacy can duplicate. The infant's breathing often settles into the cadence of the parent's chest; the parent's body, bereaved and brilliant, remembers how to soothe. A gloved finger or pacifier for non-nutritive sucking can offer powerful comfort. Mouth care with gentle swabs and balm turns a small act into a sacrament. We narrate these choices with humility: *We will keep her warm and clean and comfortable. We will protect her from unnecessary procedures.*

We will treat her body with the same reverence we did when we imagined she would live for decades.

Medicines of Mercy: Pharmacologic Ease

There are moments when non-pharmacologic tenderness is not sufficient, and pharmacology becomes the ally of love. We reach for opioids such as morphine or fentanyl when pain or air hunger threatens peace; we add a benzodiazepine when agitation or anxiety tightens the tiny limbs or creases the brow. Doses are titrated to expression, not to protocols alone: comfort shows itself in softened faces, unknotted hands, a mouth that no longer searches in distress. The intention—our moral compass—is explicit to team and family alike: we are not hastening death; we are relieving suffering. The principle is old and steady: when the aim is comfort and the means are proportional, easing distress is not only appropriate—it is required by compassion.

Secretions, the sound that troubles families the most, are addressed first by gravity and position. Side-lying and head turns allow fluid to pool where it can be wicked away; gentle suctioning avoids trauma. Anticholinergics are used sparingly when needed, explained plainly: *This may reduce the sound, though not always completely. We will watch together.* The sacred hour is a choreography of small doses and long pauses, of listening more than administering, of staying near.

The Healing Grammar of Touch, Voice, and Ritual

If one stripped neonatal end-of-life care down to its fundamental grammar, three words would remain: *touch, voice, ritual.* Touch is how mammals tell one another, "*You belong with me!*" A hand on a back, a cheek against a crown, a palm spanning the length of a torso that fits inside it—these gestures regulate heart rate and respiration, but more importantly they regulate fear. They do for the parent what they do for the child: they grant agency to arms that have felt helpless and return the body to its vocation of shelter.

Voice arrives as a second medicine. The infant's auditory world is shaped by cadence long before content. Parents who worry they "won't know what to say" discover that lullabies, whispered stories, and the simple recitation of names—grandmother, grandfather, sister, brother, dog waiting at home—become a river in which tension dissolves. The parent's voice reassures the parent as much as the child: "*I can still give something that matters.*" Reading aloud, humming, praying, or sitting in shared quiet are all forms of speech the body understands.

Ritual, finally, gives shape to the unspeakable. A bath becomes a rite of anointing; a footprint becomes a seal; a memory box becomes a reliquary. A ring slid over a wrist for a photograph becomes a family story passed to future children and grandchildren. Religious rituals—baptism, blessing, naming—are honored without rush or presumption. Secular rituals—window light, favorite song, a last walk to the unit's picture of a garden—carry equal power. What matters is meaning, not theology. The NICU team becomes, in these moments, a choir of witnesses who know how to stand still without becoming stone.

Hospice and Palliative Care: Two Lenses, One Heart

Families often ask about the difference between palliative care and hospice. In neonatology, both are languages of compassion spoken at different ranges. Palliative care begins early—at diagnosis, at delivery, at the first sign that an infant's path will be complicated. It can and should travel alongside curative intent. It is the practice of managing symptoms, clarifying values, and helping families hold the map of what lies ahead. Hospice, by contrast, centers on the last stretch of the journey, when cure has released its claim and comfort has taken the lead. In the NICU, hospice often means a thoughtful withdrawal of technology, a relocation to a family room or a home setting when possible, and an intentional weaving of memory-making into the clinical day.

Integration can take many forms. Some units adopt an integrative model: every staff member trained in primary palliative skills, from communication frameworks to symptom management, so that comfort is not a consult but a culture. Other units use a consultative model: a specialized palliative team joins when needs grow complex—difficult decisions, refractory symptoms, family dynamics that require careful tending, spiritual questions asking for presence rather than answers. In the best iterations, both models collaborate: a unit that breathes palliative values and a specialist team that can deepen and support them.

Regardless of model, the core components remain steady. Care is family-centered; parents are partners and decision-makers, not bystanders. Symptom management is expert and anticipatory, respecting that prevention is kinder than rescue. Communication is both honest and kind, unafraid of truth and unashamed of tears. For prenatal diagnoses, a birth plan articulates hopes and limits in the same breath. After death, bereavement support continues: phone calls, remembrance ceremonies, referrals, sibling support, a way to bring the hospital's promise into the family's home.

The Team That Stays Whole

If the sacred hour teaches anything, it is that clinicians must be cared for as surely as patients. Debriefs after hard cases, peer-support that is real and scheduled, and leaders who say, "take your break" and mean it—these are not luxuries; they are safeguards for the very capacities that make us worthy of the work. Compassion fatigue is the cost of porous hearts; compassion satisfaction is the dividend when systems protect those hearts. Staff rituals—speaking a baby's name at shift huddle, a butterfly on the whiteboard, a small bowl of stones placed in a jar for each life honored—give the team a way to mark what otherwise risks becoming invisible labor.

Case Vignette: Cradled in Light — A Family's Goodbye Filled with Grace

The afternoon sun arrived like a quiet benediction, slipping through the narrow NICU blinds and laying slender bands of gold across the linoleum. Nurses call it "the good light"—that hour when even the starkest rooms soften and the monitors glow like candle flames instead of command centers. On this day, the good light found **Aileen**, swaddled in lavender cotton, breathing in gentle shallow arcs, a tangle of tubing thinned at the edge of what was still needed.

Her mother, **Luz**, sat at the bedside with a braid falling over one shoulder, thumbs scrolling through photos she wasn't really seeing. **Van**, the father, stood with both palms resting on the isolette, as if feeling for a pulse in the plastic. At the foot of the bed was a small cardboard box, plain and unassuming—the kind that might hold stationery or a child's treasures. Inside: two tiny, knitted hats, a strip of paper for footprints, a miniature stethoscope charm, a vial meant for a few strands of hair. A memory box, prepared by volunteers who understand that grief needs objects to anchor it.

Dr. Tangco had spoken with them that morning, not hurried, not hedging. The words were simple and precise:

Aileen's lungs had reached their limit; her brain had been hurt by a cascade of things medicine could not undo. The team could continue to support her body with escalating technology, or they could gather around what mattered most—comfort, presence, a goodbye shaped by love. The choice felt both impossible and clear. Luz's voice trembled, but it did not break. "We want her in our arms," she said, "without the noise."

In the unit, plans for withdrawal of support are made with the same exactness afforded to resuscitations. A nurse taped a handmade sign on the curtain: **Quiet, please! Family Time.** Another dimmed the lights and silenced non-essential alarms. The respiratory therapist arranged a coil of warm tubing so it could be easily disconnected and replaced with breath that was only human. The pharmacist arrived with medications for comfort, labels tidy, intentions tender. The chaplain brought a small bowl and oil, a ribbon for blessing, and no expectation beyond presence.

All day, people moved the way we move when we do not want the floor to creak—soft-footed and attentive. Names were checked with care: Would Aileen's older brother like to be present? What song is sung at home? Are there words in another language we should know, even if only *thank you* and *peace*? The unit, so often a symphony of tasks, became liturgy.

When the hour arrived, Luz asked to bathe her daughter. Warm water was poured into a small basin. The nurse carefully lifted lines that had once been lifelines, now more like threads we were preparing to loosen. Luz washed Aileen's forehead with two fingers, then her cheeks, her soft scalp, the curve beneath her chin where milk sometimes pooled. "My girl," she whispered, "I am learning your every inch." The bath was not for cleanliness; it was for love's muscle memory. Van dried their baby with a cloth printed in constellations. "So, you'll know which stars are yours," he said, smiling the way a person smiles on a ship's deck while the sea insists on swaying.

The respiratory therapist dimmed the ventilator screen and stood close. "Whenever you're ready," she said, and waited—not for the physician's nod, but for the parents'. This is how authority should travel at the bedside: downstream from love. **Dr. Tangco** asked the team to step a pace back. "Take your time," she said. Luz lifted her daughter, wires gathered like parted vines. The ventilator was disconnected. The room exhaled.

There is an unmistakable silence that follows—the absence of the machine's tidal sigh. Aileen's chest continued its small rise and fall, as if reassured that the air between her mother's neck and shoulder was enough. A nurse slipped a tiny pulse oximeter over a toe, not to chase numbers but to notice discomfort early and relieve it before it grew teeth. The medication syringe rested in the nurse's palm, a covenant rather than a contingency.

The chaplain asked whether a blessing would be welcome. Luz nodded. The oil was unscented; the prayer was brief. "May your going be soft as light," he murmured, tracing a cross so small it could have been a star. Van placed one hand over the chaplain's and one over Luz's. "Amen," he said—a word that sometimes means *let it be so* and sometimes means, *"Help me bear what is already so."*

A child-life specialist arrived with **Gerry**, Aileen's four-year-old brother, and crouched to his height. "Would you like to meet your sister without the tubes?" she asked. He nodded. He had seen her from a distance, had learned the choreography of sanitizer and quiet voices. Now he approached, the brim of his cap bumping the isolette. "She's so tiny," he said, surprised. The nurse handed him a small, knitted cap. "Your job is to keep her warm." Gerry took the role with the gravity of knights and astronauts, touched his sister's fist with a single finger, whispered, "Hi, Lyn," trying a nickname on so the world would know he had one for her.

Photographs were taken without flash—mother and daughter cheek to cheek; father's hand spanning a whole torso; brother's hat just visible; a ring slid temporarily onto a baby's wrist so that one day, in a different season of grief, the ring could be held in a palm and the exact circumference of a life remembered. Footprints were pressed onto cardstock—one, then the other—dark blue ovals like moons. The nurse held up the card as though displaying a rare artifact. In a way, she was.

Time thickened. Breaths came further apart, then closer again, as if there were things left to smell in this world: mother's hair, father's sleeve, a cap warmed by a brother's hand. No one rushed. Medication was given in small kindnesses. **Dr. Tangco** stood at the edge of the circle, attentive without intruding, her own breath quietly syncing with Aileen's.

When the final breath arrived, it made no announcement. It simply stopped requiring the next. Luz pressed her lips to her daughter's temple and made a sound people make when sound is not enough. Van's shoulders fell and then squared again, learning in an instant the weight he would carry forever. Gerry looked up, confused by a stillness he could not name. *"Is she sleeping?"* he asked. The specialist knelt. *"She isn't hurting anymore,"* she said softly. *"She doesn't need the hospital. But we will always remember she was here."* Gerry nodded the way children do when their bodies understand more than their words.

After a while, Luz dressed Aileen in the lavender sleeper with tiny white clouds. A small lock of hair—more suggestion than strand—was placed in a vial. The footprint card dried on the counter. Someone brewed coffee and set it on a far table, then left it untouched; in grief, hospitality means not requiring anyone to drink.

Outside the curtain, the unit continued: alarms sang their thin metallic hymns; a student whispered a differential; a custodian pushed a mop with reverence learned over years. Inside the curtain, the family existed in a different tense.

"Let's take her to the window," Luz said. The good light poured itself over the sill like a blessing that never finishes. Luz swayed with the old mammalian rhythm of comfort. Van wrapped his arms around them both. Gerry pressed his face to the glass and narrated the parking lot cars—*"red, blue, silver, white."* The world, stubborn in its ordinariness, kept being the world. That felt right. That felt unbearable. That felt right.

When it was time, a nurse returned Aileen's to the bassinet, now clean of wires. *"Take as much time as you want,"* she said, and meant it. Paperwork could wait. The chaplain offered a ribbon; Luz tucked it into the memory box. The respiratory therapist, who had learned the shape of this child's breaths, placed a hand over her own heart and stepped away.

Before they left, **Dr. Tangco** asked whether they wanted one last sound: Aileen's heartbeat recorded on a small device, a keepsake to be stitched into a bear or saved as *Lyn_heart.wav.* Luz nodded. The stethoscope was warmed and placed. The rhythm's ghost was captured, then stilled. *"Thank you,"* Luz said—in grief, a sentence that means, " *You stayed with us in the hard part."*

They signed the forms. A volunteer held the elevator. The doors closed slowly, granting time for a last change of mind that never comes. Outside, cut grass and car exhaust and cafeteria fryers mixed into the smell of ordinary life. The ordinariness hurt, then helped.

Upstairs, the team gathered. *"She died in her mother's arms,"* the nurse said. *"Pain controlled." "Brother present." "Photos and footprints complete." The lavender hat goes home." "They had window light,"* the respiratory therapist added, and everyone understood how much medicine there is in light. A butterfly went up on the whiteboard beside Aileen's name—a quiet sign for soft voices and full hearts. Later, at debrief, staff spoke not to parse interventions but to honor presence.

That night, **Dr. Tangco** opened her notebook and wrote a single line: *Aileen.* Sometimes the whole entry is a name. Across town, the memory box rested on a dresser. Gerry slept with the hat under his pillow so his sister could find him in dreams. The ring Van had worn stood guard beside the box until morning.

The clinical story would eventually read like a ledger: extreme prematurity, chronic lung disease, neurologic injury, withdrawal of life support, palliative measures, death in parental arms. True, but insufficient. The truer narrative would live in the way Luz's hand curved weeks later as if still testing the size of a daughter's palm; in the way Van's shoulders squared when he said her name at counters not built for complicated answers; in the way Gerry learned to say *sister* in the past tense without apology.

What remains for the team is a sequence to be remembered and repeated: alarms softened, light invited, bath offered, pain kept small, heartbeat recorded, blessing shared, time defended, presence kept. You cannot code these acts for reimbursement. You cannot practice this work without them.

A Benediction for the Sacred Hour

The sacred hour is not a slot on a schedule; it is a stance of the heart that the unit can adopt at any time. It teaches that our task is not to engineer a perfect death—there is no such thing—but to create a trustworthy space where love is stronger than fear and gentleness outrun haste. It affirms that medicine is at its best when it knows how to stop doing and keep being, when the last intervention is to dim the light and pull up the chair.

If you return to the unit tomorrow, you may see the same sun draw the same lines across the floor. Another child will inhale new air; another will need a different kind of mercy. The sacred hour will come again, indifferent to the clock and faithful to the human need for tenderness. We will remember what we learned from Aileen and from all the children who taught us before her: that grace is not an explanation, but a way of standing with one another until the light is enough.

May we practice a medicine of soft hands and steady voices.

May our science be exact and our presence unhurried.

May every goodbye be cradled in light,

and every clinician be cradled, too.

PART III

Science, Soul, and Spirit

"Each life we touch leaves an imprint upon the soul of our practice. In every loss, we meet love in its purest form."

Arwin M. Valencia, MD

Chapter 7 – Quantum Medicine and the Energy of Connection

The Heart as a Portal

In every heartbeat lies both an electrical impulse and a whisper of intention.

Long before words are spoken or thoughts take shape, the human heart sends its rhythmic signature through the bloodstream and, more subtly, through space itself. Modern physics and neurocardiology now converge on an ancient intuition—that the heart is not merely a pump but a resonant organ of perception and communication. Its field reaches beyond the skin, weaving invisible threads between people, communities, and, perhaps, the universe itself.

Medicine has begun to acknowledge that the healing of bodies cannot be separated from the coherence of minds and hearts. Quantum biology, biofield science, and the study of electromagnetic resonance are revealing a new frontier: that connection—biological, emotional, and spiritual—is a measurable energetic phenomenon.

Coherence and Heart–Brain Resonance

The heart and brain engage in a continual dialogue. Through complex neural and biochemical pathways, each influences the other's rhythms and functions. The **"heart brain,"** composed of nearly 40000 intrinsic neurons, communicates upward through the vagus nerve more than the brain communicates downward. It sends sensory data that shape emotion, cognition, and perception.

When the rhythms of the heart and brain synchronize, a state called **physiological coherence** emerges—a measurable pattern characterized by smooth, sine-wave-like heart-rate variability. In this state, the body's major systems operate in harmony. Stress hormones subside, parasympathetic balance is restored, and cortical clarity increases. The person feels centered, peaceful, and clear-minded.

Emotions are the gatekeepers of coherence. Fear, anger, and frustration fragment heart rhythms into erratic spikes, while gratitude, compassion, and love bring order and symmetry. These shifts are not poetic metaphors—they can be charted on an electrocardiogram. Positive emotion literally reorganizes electrical information within the body.

Cultivating coherence is both art and discipline. Heart-focused breathing, meditative gratitude, mindful awareness, and prayer all entrain the cardiovascular and neural systems toward synchrony. Clinically, coherent states are linked to reduced blood pressure, improved cognitive performance, strengthened immunity, and enhanced resilience under stress. Spiritually, coherence feels like alignment—a moment when biology and being resonate as one.

Field Theory and the Unified Field

Every living system generates fields of energy. The human heart produces the largest electromagnetic field in the body—approximately **5000 times stronger** than that of the brain. Sensitive magnetometers can detect this field several feet away, suggesting that our personal space is, in truth, an interpenetrating energetic environment.

Researchers studying **interpersonal synchronization** observe that one individual's coherent heart rhythm can influence another's physiological state. Couples, parents and infants, even clinician and patient pairs show moments of synchronized heart-rate variability when empathy or shared focus arises. Such findings hint that emotional connection has a measurable energetic substrate.

Expanding further, emerging models in quantum consciousness and **biofield theory** propose that these interactions occur within a universal matrix—the **unified field** or **zero-point field**—a vast sea of energy and information underlying all physical reality. In this perspective, coherent emotion tunes human physiology to this field, facilitating intuition, creativity, and non-local connection.

When individuals or groups enter collective coherence, they may momentarily access a dimension of consciousness that transcends space and time—an experience mystics have long described as oneness.

Though these ideas remain at the edge of mainstream medicine, they challenge reductionist boundaries and invite an integrative vision: the heart as an antenna of consciousness, and love as a carrier wave of information.

The Biology of Love

Behind every feeling of closeness lies a molecular choreography dominated by **oxytocin**—a neuropeptide synthesized in the hypothalamus and released into both bloodstream and brain. Oxytocin modulates attachment, empathy, and social trust. It is secreted during childbirth, lactation, affectionate touch, and moments of emotional openness.

When oxytocin levels rise, cortisol levels fall. Heart rate slows, blood pressure stabilizes, and pain thresholds increase. This biochemical dance not only bonds mother to child or partners to one another—it fortifies immune function and fosters psychological safety. The reward system, governed by dopamine, reinforces these positive experiences, ensuring that love, comfort, and caregiving are physiologically rewarding behaviors.

Yet oxytocin is not simplistic. Context shapes its expression. Within trusted relationships it deepens empathy and cooperation, but in the presence of perceived threat it can intensify defensive loyalty to one's group. Love's biology, therefore, is not naïve sentiment—it is an adaptive strategy for connection and protection.

Bridge of Resonance

Empathy translates biology into behavior. It is the felt sense of another's interior world and forms the foundation of human compassion. Neuroimaging reveals that oxytocin heightens activity in the **insula** and **amygdala**, regions that process emotion and bodily awareness, thereby amplifying resonance with another's experience.

When a physician listens with empathy, the patient's physiology subtly shifts. Studies show lowered heart rate and blood pressure, increased vagal tone, and measurable alignment in HRV between the two individuals. In essence, empathy induces coherence not only within one person but between two—transforming a clinical encounter into a shared energetic event.

Empathy and oxytocin thus act as biological mirrors reflecting the unity implicit in human relationships. Where empathy flows, healing potential multiplies.

Intention: The Conscious Driver of Energy

If emotion harmonizes the body, **intention** directs its energy. Conscious intention—the deliberate focusing of thought and will—functions as a top-down regulatory mechanism influencing physiology and behavior. The brain's prefrontal cortex, through networks of attention and expectation, can modulate limbic and autonomic responses, effectively instructing the body how to feel and act.

Intentions shape perception. The meaning we assign to an event determines our hormonal and neural response more than the event itself. A physician who approaches a critical resuscitation with centered compassion generates a field of calm that stabilizes not only self but team and patient alike. Likewise, an anxious, fearful state transmits chaos.

Intentional practices—mindfulness, prayer, visualization, loving-kindness meditation—train these circuits. Over time, they rewire synaptic pathways, increase gray-matter density in areas related to compassion, and elevate baseline oxytocin. In quantum terms, clear intention may align personal energy with the informational currents of the unified field, amplifying outcomes that reflect coherence and care.

The Energy of Connection in Clinical Practice

In healthcare, every interaction is an exchange of energy. The clinician's emotional coherence, heart rhythm, and intention subtly influence the therapeutic environment. Patients often describe sensing "presence" or "safety" with certain caregivers even before words are spoken. These experiences mirror the phenomenon of field resonance.

When a neonatologist stands beside a fragile infant, the steadiness of breath, tone of voice, and internal coherence matter as much as pharmacology. Families feel it; infants respond to it. Quantum medicine reframes this intuitive truth into measurable dynamics of energy and information.

Training physicians to cultivate coherence—through breathing, mindfulness, or gratitude—can transform the clinical atmosphere. It restores humanity to technology-dense spaces, reminding us that healing is not imposed from the outside but evoked through relationship.

Case Vignette: "Twin Souls" — Maternal Intuition and Unexplainable Synchronicities

From her first prenatal visit, **Mrs. Valenzuela** carried an unshakable conviction that she was destined to have twins—even when every early ultrasound showed a single gestational sac. "I just know there are two," she said, resting her palms over her abdomen as if feeling twin pulses of light.

At twenty weeks, technology caught up with intuition: a second heartbeat flickered into view, hidden behind the first. Two hearts, one smaller, one strong. Tears filled her eyes. "They talk to me," she whispered.

From then on, the pregnancy unfolded like a duet. Mrs. Valenzuela could distinguish which baby was moving. When Twin A rested, she hummed low melodies; when

Twin B fluttered anxiously, she pressed her hand precisely where the smaller twin stirred. The bond felt telepathic.

At twenty-eight weeks came crisis—twin-to-twin transfusion syndrome. A delicate in-utero laser ablation was scheduled. The night before surgery, Mrs. Valenzuela dreamed of two radiant lights swirling together, one dimming as the other grew brighter until both merged into a single beam. She awoke calm, sensing meaning.

During the procedure, Twin B—the recipient—showed distress and quietly passed. Twin A's heartbeat steadied. When told the outcome, the mother nodded through tears. "He's not gone," she said softly. "He's inside his brother now."

In the NICU, the surviving twin thrived, yet uncanny patterns emerged. His monitor alarmed each night at 2:22 a.m.—the precise hour the co-twin's heart had stopped. During skin-to-skin care, when Mrs. Valenzuela whispered both names, the infant's heart rate rose whenever she spoke the lost twin's name first.

Physiologically, coincidences; symbolically, dialogue. Mrs. Valenzuela described feeling two distinct waves of milk let-down while nursing, as if feeding two. Lactation consultants confirmed the dual ejection but offered no clear explanation. Months later, she noted her son pausing mid-play to gaze into empty space, smiling as if someone unseen accompanied him.

A multidisciplinary debrief followed. The team discussed neurobiological and psychological frameworks—maternal attunement heightened by oxytocin, mirror-neuron activation, and subconscious timing cues. Yet even these could not dispel the mystery. The experience reminded every clinician that medicine and mystery are partners, not opposites.

Weeks later, a letter arrived from Mrs. Valenzuela:

> *"I no longer see two cribs, yet my heart beats in stereo.*
>
> *I feel both children when I hold one.*
>
> *Love hasn't divided—it has multiplied.*
>
> *When he laughs in his sleep, I know his brother is near."*

Closing Reflection

"Twin Souls" captures the frontier where science meets spirit. The mother's intuition, the synchronicities, and the enduring bond between her sons reveal that love is not constrained by matter. Quantum medicine offers a language for this mystery: coherence, resonance, and the unified field.

When the heart enters coherence, it becomes both transmitter and receiver of information that transcends linear time. Through empathy and intention, human beings participate in a lattice of energy that sustains life itself.

In this light, healing is no longer merely the restoration of physiology but the remembrance of connection—the realization that every cell, every heartbeat, vibrates within a universal symphony of love.

Chapter 8 – Consciousness at the Edge of Life

At the borders of birth and death, consciousness reveals its most mysterious qualities. Between the first cry of life and the last exhalation of breath lies a spectrum of awareness that transcends physiology—a subtle continuum that defies easy definition. For centuries, philosophers, mystics, and now neuroscientists have sought to understand the nature of this awareness: What happens when the brain ceases its function, yet experience continues? And could there be a deeper link between the consciousness that greets life and the one that seems to linger beyond its end?

Near-Death Experiences: The Threshold of Awareness

Near-death experiences (NDEs) are among the most compelling and enigmatic phenomena in modern medicine. They occur in moments when life itself hangs in suspension—during cardiac arrest, traumatic injury, or critical illness—when measurable brain activity ceases, yet individuals later report vivid, structured experiences.

Common features emerge across cultures and time:

- **Out-of-Body Experiences (OBEs):** A perception of floating above one's body, observing medical staff, surroundings, or even distant events with remarkable clarity.

- **The Tunnel of Light:** A sensation of movement through a dark tunnel toward an overwhelmingly radiant light—sometimes interpreted as divine or transcendent.

- **Encounters with Beings of Light:** Figures perceived as spiritual entities, ancestors, or deceased loved ones who emanate unconditional love and peace.

- **Life Review:** A panoramic replay of one's life events, often accompanied by deep insight and a profound moral or emotional evaluation of one's actions.

- **Feelings of Unity and Bliss:** A pervasive sense of oneness with all existence, an experience of infinite peace beyond human language.

To those who experience it, the NDE is not a hallucination but an encounter with ultimate reality—a moment where consciousness expands beyond biological boundaries.

From a scientific standpoint, explanations vary. Some propose that NDEs arise from anoxia (lack of oxygen), neurotransmitter surges, or temporal lobe activity during dying. Others argue that the consistency and transformative effects of these experiences—profound shifts in values, reduced fear of death, and heightened empathy—suggest that consciousness may not be fully reducible to brain activity alone.

Perinatal Awareness and the Mysteries of Beginning

Intriguingly, similar reports emerge at the other end of the life spectrum: the moment of entry into the world. "Perinatal awareness" refers to experiences or impressions associated with birth or pre-birth memory—phenomena sometimes described by children or adults under hypnosis who recall sensations of light, sound, or even emotion surrounding their own births.

Three broad categories arise:

1. **Birth Memories:** Accounts from individuals who describe the process of being born—often accompanied by feelings of compression, brightness, or relief.

2. **Perinatal Near-Death Experiences:** Mothers who have come close to death during childbirth often report the same archetypal experiences found in classical NDEs: leaving their body, seeing radiant beings, or making a choice to "return."

3. **Perinatal Trauma:** A well-documented psychological reality distinct from mystical experience, encompassing post-traumatic stress in parents following complicated deliveries or neonatal loss.

Though empirical evidence for true "birth memories" remains controversial, the recurring motifs—light, tunnel, emergence, and profound emotional resonance—mirror the symbolic language of near-death narratives.

Birth, Death, and the Mirror of Experience

In the late 20th century, psychiatrist **Stanislav Grof** and astronomer **Carl Sagan** proposed a provocative hypothesis: that NDEs might be symbolic re-enactments of the birth process. The tunnel, they suggested, represents the birth canal, the light, the entry into the world. The sense of release, love, and peace parallels the newborn's emergence from darkness into warmth and air.

Yet this "birth memory" hypothesis has been largely set aside by contemporary researchers such as **Susan Blackmore** and **Chris French**, who point out critical limitations:

- **Neurological Immaturity:** The newborn's brain lacks the cortical maturity to encode or retrieve coherent autobiographical memory.

- **C-Section NDEs:** Individuals born via cesarean section report tunnel experiences just as often as those born vaginally, undermining the birth canal analogy.

- **Affective Contrast:** The emotional tone of NDEs—serene, ecstatic, transcendent—differs radically from the stress and physiological distress of actual birth.

Nevertheless, the hypothesis opened a symbolic doorway. Even if literal birth memories are implausible, the archetypal imagery of transition—from darkness to light, confinement to expansion—may reflect universal metaphors embedded in the human psyche. Both birth and death involve surrender, transformation, and passage through an unseen threshold.

The Edge of Science: Between Empiricism and Mystery

To explore such experiences requires a rare blend of scientific rigor and philosophical humility. The limits of empirical measurement become evident when confronting phenomena that transcend the material. Consciousness itself—the medium through which all science observes—is still one of the great unsolved mysteries of existence.

Several guiding principles can illuminate the path forward:

- **Epistemic Humility:** Acknowledging that human knowledge is provisional and evolving. Science is a method of discovery, not an arbiter of ultimate truth.

- **Methodological Naturalism:** Science must remain grounded in testable hypotheses, yet this should not preclude curiosity about non-material dimensions of experience.

- **Critical Realism:** Accepting that an objective reality exists while admitting that our perception and language can only approximate it.

- **Interdisciplinary Dialogue:** Encouraging open conversations between scientists, philosophers, theologians, and those with lived experience.

Rather than viewing metaphysics as a rival to science, it may be seen as its philosophical companion—an interpretive framework that asks the deeper questions science cannot yet quantify: What is the nature of being? What sustains awareness when the brain falls silent?

Continuity of Energy and Presence

At the intersection of physics, psychology, and spirituality lies a truth that both comforts and challenges: energy never dies. According to the **Law of Conservation of Energy**, what once animated a body is transformed, not destroyed. The warmth of touch becomes heat dissipating into the air; the biochemical potential of cells returns to the earth, feeding new life.

For grieving parents, this principle can offer both scientific and spiritual solace:

- **Transformation, Not Annihilation:** The physical components of the child's body re-enter the cosmic cycle. In ashes, soil, and wind, their essence becomes part of all that is.

- **Integration with Nature:** Each molecule once part of their being continues in motion—perhaps in a breeze that touches the cheek or in the glint of morning light upon the window.

Yet the continuity extends beyond physics. The emotional and psychological connection between parent and child does not vanish at death.

- **Sensed Presence:** Many parents describe feeling their child near them—through dreams, synchronicities, or sudden waves of peace. Far from pathological, these experiences often facilitate healthy mourning and emotional integration.

- **Enduring Bond:** The attachment circuitry in the human brain does not dissolve with physical loss. Love, encoded in neural pathways, continues to generate felt connection—a form of living memory that bridges worlds.

- **Spiritual Continuity:** Across cultures, the soul or consciousness is believed to persist in a non-material dimension. Whether interpreted as energy, vibration, or divine spark, the essence of the beloved is seen as undying.

In this synthesis, science and spirituality converge. The physical world ensures continuity through transformation; the human heart ensures it through remembrance and love.

Case Vignette: "The Whisper in the Monitor" — Mystical Moments in Medicine

The Neonatal Intensive Care Unit, at night, hums with the rhythm of machines—a mechanical lullaby for the most fragile forms of life. Each beep, each wave on the monitor, marks the oscillation between existence and departure. For those who work within this sacred space, the technological and the transcendent are never far apart.

It was a quiet 3 a.m. The baby girl—born at 25 weeks—had struggled valiantly against the tide of physiology. Despite every intervention, her tiny lungs fought against the weight of immaturity. The ventilator sighed rhythmically, a mechanical breath mirroring her own dwindling effort. Around her, love filled the room like invisible light.

Her parents sat close, hands entwined beneath the soft glow of the incubator. Their eyes, red from sleepless nights, were anchored on the fragile rise and fall of her chest. The nurse, a veteran of many such nights, moved gently between them and the monitors, her gestures precise yet reverent.

Then, a subtle change. The waveforms wavered; the heart rate numbers began to drift. The room's energy shifted into a profound stillness—a moment suspended outside of time. The nurse later described it as a "presence," something ineffable that filled the air.

The mother leaned closer, whispering, "It's okay, my love. You can rest now. We'll always be with you." Her words trembled through tears, yet carried a strange serenity. The father reached inside the incubator, his fingertip brushing his daughter's palm.

And then, the monitor sang.

For a brief, astonishing instant, the rhythmic beeps aligned into a pattern—a sequence of tones forming what all present described as a melody. It was delicate, like a lullaby—three soft notes rising, then falling. The nurse froze, her breath catching. The parents looked at each other, disbelief and awe mingling. "Did you hear that?" the mother whispered. "She's saying goodbye," murmured the father.

Moments later, the heart rate line flattened into silence.

The air did not grow heavy with despair. Instead, it seemed to lighten—as if the room itself exhaled. The nurse felt tears well, not from sorrow alone, but from something luminous—a peace too vast for words.

When the data were later reviewed, the melody could not be explained. The monitor's alarm logs showed no such pattern. It was, by all technical accounts, impossible. And yet, for those who witnessed it, it was as real as touch, as sacred as prayer.

In that moment, medicine bowed before mystery.

Reflection: Science and the Soul's Horizon

Such stories defy categorization. Were they coincidences born of grief and heightened perception? Or glimpses of a consciousness that extends beyond the brain's circuitry?

For the clinician, these moments challenge the boundaries of training. Medicine teaches us to measure—to quantify and categorize—but at the threshold of life and death, we encounter something unmeasurable. The physician becomes both witness and pilgrim, standing at the altar of the unknown.

Perhaps the deeper question is not whether these events are *real* in a physical sense, but what they reveal about the nature of love and consciousness itself. If consciousness is not confined to the body, then perhaps every act of compassion, every word spoken in farewell, becomes a thread in the vast fabric of being—vibrations that continue to resonate in unseen dimensions.

In this way, the Neonatal Intensive Care Unit becomes more than a ward of medicine—it becomes a sanctuary of mystery. The beeps of the monitor are not merely data points but hymns of existence; the pauses between them, the silence of the infinite.

Closing Reflection: The Circle of Light

Birth and death are not opposites, but reflections—each a portal through which consciousness transitions between forms. The same light that welcomes the newborn at first breath may be the one that receives the soul at its final sigh.

Perhaps consciousness, like energy, cannot be destroyed—only transformed. It flickers between dimensions, whispering through monitors, breathing through parents' tears, glowing through the memories that refuse to fade.

In honoring these thresholds, medicine fulfills its highest calling: not merely to sustain biological life, but to recognize and reverence the sacred continuity of being. Between the first heartbeat and the last lies the mystery of consciousness—a light that neither begins nor ends, but forever illumines the edge of life.

Chapter 9 – Healing Through Meaning

Healing after loss is not the same as forgetting, and meaning is not found by escaping pain, but by transforming it. In the NICU, where life begins at the threshold of fragility, caregivers and families encounter daily the profound paradox of human existence—where love and suffering coexist, where science and spirit intertwine, and where the search for meaning becomes the most vital form of healing.

At the heart of this search stands the work of Viktor Frankl, an Austrian psychiatrist and Holocaust survivor, whose **logotherapy** emerged as a beacon for those seeking purpose amid suffering. Frankl taught that even when everything else is taken from us, the last of human freedoms remains: the ability to choose one's attitude toward any given circumstance. His insight, born from unimaginable loss, offers a powerful framework for parents, families, and clinicians facing grief within the NICU.

Logotherapy and the Search for Meaning

Frankl's **logotherapy** is rooted in the premise that the deepest human drive is not pleasure or power—but meaning. Through meaning, suffering can be transformed from a source of despair into an instrument of growth.

He identified what he called the **"tragic triad"**—*pain, guilt,* and *death*—as inescapable realities of human existence. Yet within this triad lies the potential for transcendence. Pain can reveal courage; guilt can call forth growth; death can awaken love and urgency to live more fully.

The Power of Attitude

Frankl proposed that no matter how limited one's circumstances, there always remains one final freedom: to choose one's response. Even in the face of unbearable loss—such as the death of a child—an individual can cultivate an attitude that gives the suffering meaning.

One bereaved father, for instance, once told Frankl that he had chosen to bear his suffering as a way of sparing his son future pain. That conscious reframes transformed grief into a selfless act of love. Likewise, many NICU parents find meaning not by escaping sorrow, but by transforming it into compassion, advocacy, or service to others.

Meaning Through Creation, Experience, and Responsibility

Frankl identified three primary pathways to meaning:

- **Through creation:** By bringing something into the world—be it art, a deed, or a project—we transcend suffering through creative purpose.

- **Through experience:** By opening ourselves to love, nature, beauty, or spiritual wonder, we experience meaning directly.

- **Through attitude:** When faced with unavoidable suffering, we can still choose how we respond, giving purpose to pain by aligning it with our deepest values.

Ultimately, meaning is not found in what happens to us, but in what we make of what happens.

Suffering as a Catalyst for Transformation

Frankl never glorified suffering. Logotherapy emphasizes that meaning is possible *in spite of* suffering—not *because of* it. Unavoidable pain can become an opportunity for transformation, but if suffering can be prevented or alleviated, compassion demands that it should be.

In neonatal care, this distinction is critical. Medical teams strive to relieve suffering whenever possible, yet when death cannot be averted, the work shifts from *curing* to *caring*, from preserving life to preserving meaning.

For many families, this shift begins in the sacred space between heartbreak and grace—where surrender, remembrance, and meaning converge.

Spiritual Resilience and the Art of Surrender

Spiritual resilience is the capacity to maintain a sense of self, purpose, and faith amid adversity. It is not about denial of pain, but about drawing strength from one's inner beliefs and values.

At its core lies the **art of surrender**—not as passive resignation, but as a courageous act of trust. Surrender invites acceptance: to stop resisting what cannot be changed, and to discover peace in the midst of uncertainty.

The Link Between Surrender and Resilience

- **Releasing Control:** Much of human suffering stems from the illusion of control. In the NICU, where life hangs by threads of probability, surrender becomes an act of freedom—allowing parents and caregivers to redirect energy from anxiety toward presence and love.

- **Acceptance as Flow:** Acceptance allows one to move with life's current instead of against it, fostering emotional flexibility—the very essence of resilience.

- **Faith in the Unseen:** Many parents speak of surrendering their child into divine hands, believing that life continues in a higher dimension. This faith sustains them when logic fails.

- **Opening to New Possibilities:** When attachment to specific outcomes softens, new insights, creative expressions, and acts of meaning-making emerge—what Frankl might call "defiant power of the human spirit."

- **Healing Through Letting Go:** Releasing guilt, anger, and helplessness becomes the doorway to emotional freedom and post-traumatic growth.

Through surrender, suffering becomes not an endpoint, but a passageway—one that deepens empathy, broadens perspective, and reconnects the heart to the sacred rhythm of life.

Rituals of Remembrance in the NICU

Grief rituals, journaling, and memorialization are not mere sentimental gestures; they are **sacred technologies of meaning**. They help families reclaim a sense of agency, integrate their loss into the narrative of love, and affirm that every life—no matter how brief—matters profoundly.

Grief Rituals

Hospitals have begun to incorporate family-centered rituals that honor both medical reality and emotional truth:

- **Holding and Touching:** Parents are encouraged to hold their infant, even after death. The tactile memory of warmth and weight becomes a vital link between the physical and the eternal.

- **Bathing and Dressing:** Parents may bathe and dress their baby in "angel gowns" or personal clothing—continuing the act of parenting through ritual care.

- **Cultural and Religious Ceremonies:** Baptisms, blessings, and dedications are facilitated to bring spiritual closure in alignment with the family's faith.

- **Naming the Baby:** A name gives the child identity and recognition; it affirms that they were, and always will be, part of the family story.

- **Private Farewell:** Families are offered time to say goodbye in peace, away from the hum of machines, within an atmosphere of reverence.

These small yet sacred acts anchor grief in love, transforming a sterile environment into holy ground.

Journaling and the Written Heart

Journaling serves as a mirror to the soul, a safe container where parents can express raw emotion and begin to reweave the threads of their shattered world.

- **Emotional Release:** Writing helps articulate pain that cannot be spoken aloud.

- **Preserving Memory:** Each entry becomes a testimony of love, a diary of moments that affirm the baby's existence.

- **Restoring Agency:** In a world of medical uncertainty, journaling offers a small realm of control and authorship.

- **Creating Legacy:** Over time, the journal evolves into a keepsake—a love story written in ink and tears.

In some NICUs, nurses add their reflections, turning these journals into shared testaments of compassion, connection, and remembrance.

Memorialization and Keepsakes

For families leaving the NICU without their child, tangible keepsakes become symbols of continuity.

Memory boxes often include:

- Handprints or footprints cast in plaster
- A lock of hair
- ID bracelets and crib cards
- Photographs taken by compassionate staff
- A blanket or hat worn by the baby
- Notes and poems from caregivers

Outside the hospital, families may extend these memorials by planting trees, crafting jewelry with tiny footprints, lighting candles on anniversaries, or creating living memorials, like Tina and Jamil's *"Grace's Garden"*, a story of grief transfigured into beauty.

Case Vignette: Grace's Garden: Tina and Jamil's Journey of Transforming Pain into Legacy

Grace was born at twenty-four weeks, a wisp of life weighing barely over a pound. Her skin was translucent, her heartbeat fragile, her breath sustained by rhythm and light. Every sound in the Neonatal Intensive Care Unit (NICU), beeping monitors, ventilator sighs, seemed to harmonize with her will to survive.

Her parents, **Tina** and **Jamil,** hovered beside her isolette, whispering lullabies through tears. "We named her Grace," Tina said softly, "because we knew we would need it."

The Fragile Beginning

From her first moments, Grace lived in a delicate balance between science and spirit. The medical team acted with precision and reverence—intubating, adjusting, monitoring—while knowing that outcomes lay beyond control. Each sunrise that followed was received not as a guarantee, but as a gift.

The Crossroads of Hope and Sorrow

Weeks passed. Grace endured infections, bradycardias, and procedures with quiet strength. Her small hand would sometimes curl around her mother's finger, anchoring Tina's hope. Yet as her lungs weakened, the inevitable conversation came. "If we let her go," Tina whispered, "will she suffer?" The neonatologist replied, "We will make sure her final moments are filled only with love."

The Sacred Hour

When the machines were silenced, Grace was placed in her mother's arms—finally free of tubes and wires. Skin met skin, heart met heart. Jamil held them both as the monitor traced one last rhythm before fading into stillness. Time itself seemed to pause. The room, though silent, vibrated with something eternal—love distilled to its purest form.

From Grief to Growth

In the weeks that followed, Tina wandered through a fog of sorrow until one afternoon she felt compelled to work the earth in her backyard. She began to plant—lilies, forget-me-nots, white roses. Each bloom, she said, was "a prayer made visible."

Thus, *Grace's Garden* was born. What began as a mother's personal ritual of healing became a sanctuary for others. Bereaved parents soon came to plant their own flowers, each representing a story of love that had briefly touched the earth.

The Garden as Legacy

Over time, *Grace's Garden* grew into a living memorial—hosting remembrance ceremonies and vigils. Nurses came on their days off to reflect and reconnect with purpose. The neonatologist began bringing new fellows there, saying, "This is where medicine meets meaning."

Jamil installed a gentle fountain at the center, the water's whisper symbolizing continuity—the heartbeat they could no longer hear, but still felt.

The Transmutation of Sorrow

Grace's Garden stands today as a testament that grief, when tended with compassion, becomes fertile soil for healing. It embodies Frankl's wisdom that even amidst the tragic triad of pain, guilt, and death, there remains an unbroken thread of meaning.

For Tina and Jamil, their daughter's brief life continues to bloom in every flower and every parent who finds solace there. Each anniversary, Tina writes:

> *"We planted a garden not to bury our sorrow,*
>
> *but to let it bloom into light.*
>
> *In every petal, she breathes anew,*
>
> *our little Grace, forever growing."*

Healing through meaning does not erase suffering—it transforms it. In the sacred space of the NICU, where medicine meets mystery, every act of remembrance, surrender, and love becomes a seed. From these seeds, gardens of grace arise—proof that from the deepest pain, the human spirit can still create beauty, connection, and eternal life.

PART IV

Integration and Transformation

Chapter 10 - Building a Culture of Compassionate Care

The Neonatal Intensive Care Unit (NICU) is more than a medical environment — it is a crucible of human emotion, where grief and gratitude, fragility and resilience, coexist in a delicate equilibrium. The staff who serve in this space bear witness to both the beginning and end of life, often within the same shift. Over time, this exposure to profound human suffering can leave invisible scars unless organizations intentionally create systems that protect and nourish the caregivers themselves.

To build a culture of compassionate care, institutions must integrate *policies that protect, resources that sustain, and practices that heal.* These elements form the scaffolding for a resilient, empathetic, and ethically grounded healthcare community.

1. Clear and Inclusive Bereavement Leave Policies

Compassionate care begins not only at the bedside but also within the organization's structure. A transparent and humane bereavement policy communicates one vital message: *your humanity is valued here.*

- **Eligibility and Duration**: Policies should specify who qualifies (full-time, part-time, or contract employees) and outline the length of leave — typically three to five days for immediate family, though progressive institutions now offer up to twenty days with flexibility to accommodate individual circumstances.

- **Inclusive Family Definitions**: The modern understanding of family extends beyond biological ties. Policies should recognize domestic partners, chosen family, and close friends, and explicitly include pregnancy loss, miscarriage, and stillbirth.

- **Flexibility and Humanity**: Grief does not conform to a schedule. Allowing non-consecutive leave days or phased returns can ease reentry. Options for remote work, adjusted workloads, or additional unpaid leave can provide crucial space for emotional healing.

- **Compassion over Bureaucracy**: Unless mandated, documentation such as death certificates should not be required. Compassionate policies trust the employee's integrity and prioritize empathy over proof.

- **Communication and Accessibility:** Policies must be easy to find, clearly written, and accompanied by a designated contact person (often HR or a wellness liaison) to guide the grieving employee through the process.

A well-crafted bereavement policy affirms that compassion is not just a bedside virtue — it is an institutional standard.

2. Access to Emotional Support Resources

Time off alone cannot mend a broken heart. Healing also requires access to emotional and psychological support systems designed to restore balance and resilience.

- **Employee Assistance Programs (EAPs):** Confidential counseling, financial, and legal guidance offered to staff, and their families can serve as a first line of emotional support.

- **Specialized Grief Counseling:** Institutions should ensure mental health coverage includes counselors trained in perinatal grief, trauma, and loss.

- **Support Groups:** Facilitated peer groups, whether in person or virtual, provide connection and shared understanding among those who have endured similar losses.

- **Managerial and Peer Training:** Supervisors and HR staff must be educated in bereavement sensitivity, recognizing signs of complicated grief, and fostering open dialogue.

A culture of care thrives when support is visible, accessible, and normalized — when seeking help is seen as strength, not stigma.

3. Supportive Workplace Culture and Practical Compassion

Policies and programs are only effective if they are embodied through everyday compassion. Healing culture is built not in mission statements but in moments of human connection.

- **Acknowledge the Loss:** Silence can unintentionally wound. Simple, sincere words — "I'm so sorry for your loss" — often mean more than polished condolences.

- **Offer Tangible Help:** Replace open-ended offers ("Let me know if you need anything") with specific actions ("I'll cover your shift on Tuesday" or "I'll handle the rounds this morning").

- **Respect Privacy and Boundaries:** Allow individuals to decide how much of their story to share and when. Avoid contacting them about work matters during their bereavement period.

- **Facilitate a Gentle Return**: Create a phased reintegration plan with regular check-ins and flexible expectations.

- **Memorialize with Sensitivity**: When a staff member passes, institutions can coordinate memorial gestures — such as planting a tree, dedicating a space, or making a donation — always in consultation with the family.

The essence of compassionate culture is not grand gestures but consistency — the quiet, ongoing reassurance that *you are not alone.*

4. Institutional Healing Mechanisms: Debriefings, Peer Support, and Trauma-Informed Systems

Healthcare professionals are both healers and humans. The cumulative effect of repeated exposure to suffering can lead to compassion fatigue, burnout, and secondary trauma. Institutions that wish to preserve the heart of their workforce must embed healing practices into their daily rhythm.

Team Debriefings

Debriefings are structured, restorative dialogues held soon after a critical event — such as a patient death or ethical dilemma — allowing team members to process emotions, share perspectives, and reinforce psychological safety.

- **Timing**: Conducted within 24–48 hours of the incident to ensure immediacy and emotional clarity.

- **Safe Space**: A private, non-judgmental environment where hierarchy dissolves and honesty is invited.

- **Facilitation**: Led by a trained moderator (e.g., psychologist, chaplain, or senior nurse) who promotes open sharing rather than performance evaluation.

- **Content**: Focused on three reflective questions — *What went well? What didn't? What can we do differently next time?*

- **Follow-Up**: Documenting lessons learned and assigning actionable improvements reinforces growth and trust.

Debriefings remind the team that vulnerability is not a liability; it is the birthplace of collective wisdom.

Peer Counseling and Peer Support

Sometimes, the most effective form of healing comes from someone who truly understands.

- **Role and Scope:** Peer counselors offer confidential, non-clinical emotional support grounded in empathy and shared experience.

- **Training and Selection:** Volunteers are chosen for emotional maturity and trained in active listening, boundaries, and psychological first aid.

- **Trust and Confidentiality:** Trust is the cornerstone — conversations remain confidential unless safety is at risk.

- **Integration into Culture:** Peer programs must be supported by leadership and integrated into broader wellness initiatives, ensuring accessibility and sustainability.

When peers listen without judgment, the isolation of grief gives way to solidarity.

Trauma-Informed Systems

A trauma-informed organization recognizes that trauma, whether from personal loss, workplace stress, or exposure to suffering — affects how people think, feel, and work. Its framework is built on the **"Four R's":**

1. **Realize** the widespread impact of trauma.

2. **Recognize** its signs in individuals and systems.

3. **Respond** by weaving trauma awareness into daily practice.

4. **Resist re-traumatization** through conscious policies and behaviors.

Core principles include safety, trust, peer support, collaboration, empowerment, and cultural awareness.

Leaders must model empathy, prioritize staff well-being, and replace "What's wrong with you?" with "What happened to you?"

By aligning administrative compassion with emotional literacy, trauma-informed systems transform institutions from places of performance into sanctuaries of healing.

Case Vignette: "The Team That Cried Together" — Collective Healing After Loss

The call came just before dawn. The monitors' alarms, once our rhythm of reassurance, now echoed in dissonance — sharp reminders of a fragile life slipping away. Despite every effort, every ounce of skill and prayer, the baby's tiny heart could not be persuaded to stay. When the monitor flatlined, so did the unspoken hope that had bound us together through the long night.

In the silence that followed, the room held its breath. The nurse who had gently cradled the baby's hand withdrew her gloved fingers, tears filling her eyes. The respiratory therapist leaned back, his hands trembling slightly as he shut down the ventilator. A resident whispered, "Time of death, 4:27 a.m." Her voice cracked under the weight of the moment. No one moved for a while — as if any motion might shatter the sacred stillness that had settled between us.

The Shared Burden of Compassion

The NICU is a place where science and spirit meet in fragile balance. We celebrate miracles measured in grams and millimeters, yet face tragedies that defy even the best technology. For the care team, each loss is not just a medical outcome but a human rupture — a quiet wound that lingers behind the sterile precision of our tasks.

That morning, none of us left the bedside immediately. Instead, we stayed — some standing, others sitting — surrounding the tiny body as if to shield it from the coldness of the world. The mother's sobs filled the space, raw and holy. A nurse placed the baby gently in her arms, wrapped in a white blanket with a blue and pink ribbon. "Take all the time you need," she whispered. We stepped back, hands clasped, heads bowed. It wasn't protocol. It was reverence.

When the Healers Need Healing

After the family left, the hum of machinery resumed, but the emotional weight lingered. During the morning huddle, silence stretched long until a nurse whispered, "It feels like we failed." Another responded, "We did everything, but sometimes everything isn't enough." The attending physician looked around the room and said quietly, "We cry because we care. If we ever stop crying, that's when we should worry."

Tears broke the barrier of professionalism. For once, we allowed ourselves to grieve together — not in isolation, but in communion.

Rituals of Remembrance

In the weeks that followed, the unit decided to honor losses more openly. We began placing a white origami butterfly in a glass jar each time a baby passed. Once a month, the team gathered for a moment of remembrance — sometimes silent, sometimes prayerful. One nurse said softly, "I used to think tears made me weak. Now I think they make me whole."

We shared not just sorrow but gratitude — stories of parents who sang lullabies through tears, fathers who whispered thanks for brief but infinite love. These moments became our medicine, restoring meaning where reason faltered.

From Compassion Fatigue to Compassion Renewal

Healthcare often speaks of *compassion fatigue,* but this experience revealed something deeper — *compassion renewal.* When grief is shared, it transforms from burden to bond.

The social worker began hosting regular reflective sessions, offering a sacred pause amid clinical busyness. Slowly, the culture shifted from "getting through" to "healing through." Emotional expression became a mark of integrity, not weakness — a vital sign of the soul.

The Unspoken Bond

Months later, another fragile infant teetered between life and loss. When the outcome turned grim, a nurse reached for her colleague's hand and said, "Whatever happens, we'll face it together." That sentence carried the resonance of healing — not the kind measured by survival, but by solidarity.

In the NICU, where beginnings and endings intertwine, the team learned that healing does not always mean saving a life. Sometimes, it means saving *each other* — through shared tears, silent prayers, and the collective courage to keep showing up.

Each butterfly added to the jar became a symbol of both memory and transformation — not only for the children we lost but for the team that rediscovered its heart through grief shared and compassion renewed.

Chapter 11 – Lessons from the Light

The Neonatal Intensive Care Unit (NICU) is more than a medical environment—it is a sacred classroom where the lessons of love, loss, and transcendence unfold daily. Within its softly humming machines, flickering monitors, and quiet prayers whispered through tears, life's most profound truths are revealed. It is a place where science meets spirit, and where the fragile boundary between life and death becomes a teacher in compassion, humility, and grace.

A Sacred Classroom

To call the NICU a "sacred classroom" is to acknowledge that it is a space of awakening. Here, parents and caregivers are invited to witness the mystery of life stripped bare of illusion—where every breath, every heartbeat, every tiny movement carries infinite weight.

The sterile walls of the unit, though clinical in appearance, hold an atmosphere that transcends the ordinary. Within them, love and fear coexist. Time feels suspended, and the smallest changes—a rise in oxygen saturation, a soft cry, a parent's touch—become monumental.

In this classroom, the students are not just the physicians, nurses, or parents, they are souls learning to expand through vulnerability, faith, and surrender. The lessons are not written in textbooks, but in the lived experiences of those who stand at the threshold between beginnings and endings.

Lessons of Love

At the heart of the NICU lies an unspoken truth: love heals in ways medicine alone cannot.

Parents discover a form of love so raw and unconditioned that it defies circumstance. It is love that shows up through exhaustion, fear, and hope; love that speaks through touch when words fail; love that persists even in silence.

- **Connection Heals:** Skin-to-skin contact, known as kangaroo care, is more than a therapeutic intervention—it is communion. The rhythm of a parent's heartbeat steadies the infant's. The warmth of touch becomes medicine for both, fostering regulation, growth, and deep emotional bonding.

- **Unconditional Love:** Amid ventilators and IV lines, parents learn to see beyond diagnoses and prognosis. They love not for potential, but for presence—for the sacredness of *this moment*, however uncertain.

- **Vulnerability as Strength:** Love in the NICU teaches courage—the courage to trust strangers with your child's life, to ask for help, and to surrender control. True strength emerges not from holding on, but from opening one's heart to the unknown.

Every act of love—be it a nurse's gentle repositioning of a tiny arm, or a mother's whispered lullaby through tears—becomes an offering to life itself.

Lessons of Loss

Loss in the NICU takes many forms. It is not confined to death, though that shadow sometimes visits. It is the loss of expectations, the imagined normalcy of birth, the simple joys of holding a baby without monitors or alarms. It is grief intertwined with hope—an emotional paradox that families and caregivers learn to navigate together.

- **Grief in Many Forms:** Parents grieve the birth they didn't have, the milestones delayed or missed, the uncertain tomorrows. Staff grieve too—quietly, collectively, carrying the memory of every tiny hand they've ever held.

- **Honoring Life, However Brief:** Even when life lasts only moments or days, it holds immeasurable meaning. These infants, in their brevity, teach depth—showing that love's measure is not in duration, but in presence. Nurses, physicians, and chaplains learn to honor these sacred hours, bearing witness to the holiness of beginnings and endings intertwined.

- **Redefining Hope:** Hope in the NICU transforms. It is no longer confined to the outcome of survival but expands into gratitude for each small victory—a stable vital sign, a first feeding, a moment of peace. Hope becomes a spiritual resilience, a light that endures even when the path is unclear.

Through loss, the NICU teaches reverence. It reminds all who enter that every soul—no matter how brief its stay—leaves an indelible mark on the hearts it touches.

Lessons of Transcendence

Transcendence in the NICU is the quiet miracle that arises from suffering transformed into meaning. It is the shift from, *"Why this happened?"* to *"What can this teach me?"* from despair to purpose, from brokenness to awakening.

- **Finding Purpose:** Many parents and caregivers channel their pain into service. They return to advocate, to support, to comfort others walking the same uncertain road. Their grief becomes a catalyst for healing beyond themselves.

- **Perspective and Priorities:** Within the NICU, the trivial dissolves. What once seemed urgent—emails, deadlines, daily stress—fades in the presence of a fragile breath. The experience realigns priorities, deepening appreciation for the simple miracles of family, health, and time.

- **Spiritual Awakening:** The proximity to life and death invites profound contemplation. Some rediscover faith; others find spirituality beyond religion—a quiet knowing that love transcends form, and that every soul, no matter how small, participates in something eternal.

Through transcendence, the NICU becomes more than a place of healing for infants—it becomes a sanctuary for human evolution, where science and spirit merge in the shared pursuit of compassion.

The Eternal Lesson

In this sacred classroom, fragility and strength are not opposites—they coexist. The NICU reminds us that healing does not always mean cure, and that presence itself can be the highest form of medicine. For those who have walked its halls, the lessons endure long after discharge or farewell: to love without condition, to grieve without shame, and to find meaning in every breath.

The NICU is, indeed, a holy teacher—one that humbles, transforms, and awakens all who listen to its quiet wisdom.

Chapter 12 – The Light Endures

Integrating **science, soul, and sanctity** in modern medicine represents a long-awaited reunion between empirical knowledge and the wisdom of the human spirit. This union invites clinicians, families, and patients alike to approach healing as a multidimensional process—one that honors the intricate physiology of the body while also tending to the unseen dimensions of emotion, meaning, and faith. Within the Neonatal Intensive Care Unit (NICU), where fragile beginnings and uncertain outcomes coexist, this integration becomes both an ethical necessity and a sacred calling.

Science Meets the Sacred

Modern medicine has advanced at a breathtaking pace, decoding the genetic and cellular foundations of life. Yet even amid these triumphs of knowledge, an unspoken truth lingers: science, without soul, can become mechanical; treatment, without tenderness, incomplete. Healing transcends the mere alleviation of symptoms—it touches the human need for connection, understanding, and hope.

In recent decades, research has begun to validate what caregivers have intuitively known for centuries: that **spirituality and meaning-making are integral to health.** Studies conducted by institutions such as Harvard and the National Institutes of Health reveal measurable benefits associated with spiritual engagement—lower stress levels, improved immune response, enhanced coping in chronic illness, and greater patient satisfaction. These findings affirm that compassion and presence are not peripheral gestures, but active ingredients in healing.

The Essence of Whole-Person Care

Spirituality, in this context, is not confined to religion. It is the universal human quest to find purpose, belonging, and transcendence. For some, it may emerge through faith traditions, for others, through nature, love, art, or service. To integrate spirituality into medicine, then, is to **treat the person rather than the pathology**, to see each patient not as a diagnosis but as a soul in evolution.

Whole-person care demands that we move beyond the fragmented model that separates mind from body, and body from spirit. It calls for a holistic view—one that recognizes how emotions influence physiology, how beliefs shape recovery, and how connection fosters resilience. In the NICU, this approach takes on profound meaning. Here, a mother's touch, a father's whispered prayer, or a nurse's gentle lullaby may carry as much healing power as any medication or intervention.

Pathways to Integration

Integrating spirituality into clinical practice is both an art and a discipline. Several methods have proven effective in bridging this once-imagined divide between medicine and meaning:

- **Spiritual History-Taking:** Just as we inquire about family history or medications, clinicians can ask brief, compassionate questions about a patient's beliefs or sources of strength. A simple inquiry such as, *"What gives you hope?"* can open a doorway to understanding the patient's deeper needs.

- **Interprofessional Collaboration:** Chaplains, pastoral care providers, and spiritual counselors can be vital members of the healthcare team. Their presence ensures that care remains compassionate even in moments of profound suffering, allowing the sacred dimension of healing to be acknowledged and supported.

- **Clinician Training:** Programs that teach physicians and nurses how to address spirituality with respect and sensitivity are growing. Training fosters humility, empathy, and awareness—qualities essential to healing professions that deal daily with life, loss, and the mystery between.

- **Mind–Body Practices:** Integrative modalities such as mindfulness, yoga, acupuncture, and meditation are not merely complementary but evidence-based. They reduce stress hormones, improve heart rate variability, and promote a state of physiological coherence—aligning body rhythms with emotional balance.

- **Patient-Centered Communication:** At its heart, spiritual care requires presence. When a clinician listens deeply, with genuine compassion, healing begins—sometimes even before treatment is administered.

Challenges and Opportunities

Despite growing recognition, obstacles remain. Many healthcare systems still prioritize efficiency over empathy, constrained by time, documentation, and the pressure of outcomes. Few clinicians receive formal training in addressing the spiritual dimension, and some hesitate for fear of overstepping boundaries.

Yet opportunities abound. The emergence of initiatives such as the **NIH Religion, Spirituality, and Health Scientific Interest Group** signals a paradigm shift. Institutions are beginning to explore integrative frameworks that unite scientific rigor with spiritual understanding. This evolution reflects an acknowledgment that the human being is not a sum of organs, but a living synthesis of body, mind, and spirit.

If medicine is to be truly modern, it must also be timeless—anchored in compassion, guided by evidence, and illuminated by the enduring truth that **healing begins when we see the sacred in one another.**

The Spiritual Physiology of Hope

Hope, like breath, sustains life. It is not a passive wish, but an active energy—a biological, psychological, and spiritual force that propels the will to survive and the courage to endure. In the NICU, where uncertainty is constant, hope functions as both medicine and miracle.

Scientific studies show that hope alters physiology. It reduces cortisol, the hormone of stress, while enhancing immune and cardiovascular function. The brain, when hopeful, releases endorphins and dopamine—chemicals that lessen pain and amplify motivation. But beyond its neurobiology, hope holds a sacred dimension: it anchors the soul in the conviction that life, however fragile, is meaningful.

The Anatomy of Hope

Hope exists on two levels:

- **Internal**—rooted in self-worth and agency, the belief that one can act toward healing.

- **External**—grounded in faith, trust, or surrender to something greater than oneself.

When these two dimensions converge, hope becomes a living bridge between the known and the unknown, between science and spirit. It embodies both **agency**—the determination to act—and **faith**—the belief that one's efforts are supported by divine or universal grace.

Physiological and Psychological Effects

- **Stress Reduction:** Hope lowers sympathetic activation, calming the body's fight-or-flight response.

- **Pain Modulation:** Expectation and belief trigger the release of natural pain-relieving neurochemicals.

- **Immunity and Recovery:** Hopeful patients demonstrate stronger immune responses and faster healing.

- **Resilience:** Hope reframes suffering, allowing individuals to find meaning even in adversity.

Cultivating Hope in Practice

Hope is cultivated through both attitude and ritual. It grows in the soil of **faith, patience, and courage**. It is sustained through **connection, meaning, and storytelling**. In the NICU, rituals of hope may include lighting a candle, writing a letter to a child, or simply sitting in silence beside an incubator, whispering love into the unseen spaces.

- **Spiritual Beliefs and Practices:** Prayer, meditation, and sacred music can restore inner equilibrium and strengthen one's sense of trust.

- **Visualization and Intention:** Imagining healing and writing affirmations of gratitude help direct the mind toward possibility.

- **Mindful Reflection:** Gentle self-inquiry—asking "What gives my life meaning?"—reconnects the heart to purpose.

- **Patience and Persistence:** True hope endures delays and setbacks, seeing beyond the moment into the mystery of unfolding grace.

In the presence of such hope, even the smallest victories—an infant's stable heartbeat, a parent's first touch, a caregiver's quiet prayer—become holy milestones.

161

Healing Beyond Cure

There are moments in medicine when cure is not possible, yet healing still occurs. This paradox defines much of neonatal care. Families who face the loss of a newborn encounter depths of sorrow few can comprehend, yet within that sorrow often arises an awakening: a recognition that love transcends mortality.

Healing, in this sense, is not the erasure of pain but its transformation. It is the alchemy through which grief becomes gratitude, despair becomes faith, and memory becomes light. The role of the caregiver extends beyond technical expertise—it becomes a ministry of presence. By holding space for both life and death, clinicians participate in the sacred rhythm of existence itself.

Closing Reflections: "Every Life—No Matter How Brief—Illuminates Eternity"

In the quiet hum of the Neonatal Intensive Care Unit, where time often feels suspended between a heartbeat and a breath, we are reminded that the measure of a life cannot be captured in minutes, days, or even years. Each tiny soul, whether they stay for an instant or a season, leaves an imprint that transcends the boundaries of time. Their existence, brief as it may appear, becomes an eternal light that guides those who remain.

Every life is a spark of the Infinite—a reflection of divine intention. These infants, fragile yet luminous, come into our care as living reminders that love itself is eternal. They awaken in us a sacred awareness: that even the smallest heartbeat carries infinite meaning, and even the briefest encounter can change the trajectory of a life. Through them, we witness not only the delicate balance of physiology but also the boundless mystery of spirit.

Families who walk through the valley of loss emerge transformed. In their grief, they discover the depths of love's endurance. They learn that to have held a child, even for a fleeting moment, is to have touched eternity. Nurses, physicians, and caregivers, too, are changed by these encounters. In tending to fragile lives, they become stewards of light—guardians of both life and legacy.

The NICU, then, is not merely a place of medicine but of meaning. Within its walls, science and soul intertwine. It becomes a sacred classroom where the lesson is love, the curriculum is compassion, and the final revelation is that no life is ever truly lost. Each heartbeat, however brief, sends ripples through eternity—echoes of courage, tenderness, and divine connection that continue long after the monitors fall silent.

And so, as we close this reflection, we return to the truth that has guided every chapter of this journey: **Every life— no matter how brief—illuminates eternity.** In the flicker of each newborn's light, we glimpse the timeless essence of existence itself—a radiant reminder that love is the only force that never fades.

Epilogue — Love Beyond Measure

In the hush between heartbeats, a story unfolds,
not written in ink, but in pulse and breath.
A mother's whisper meets a child's sigh,
and time, for a moment, stands still.

Here in this sacred circle,
the healer kneels beside the cradle of beginnings,
hands steady, spirit trembling,
aware that the work is not only to mend, but to witness.

The child, small as a prayer, speaks without words:
"Love me as I am, not for how long I stay."

And so, the parents do,
with eyes that memorize every rise of the chest,
every flicker of light through translucent skin,
their souls expanding beyond the boundaries
of flesh and fear.

The healer listens too,
to monitors that hum like distant choirs,
to silence that feels holy,
to the unseen dialogue between soul and soul.

In that exchange, something eternal stirs:
a remembrance that medicine, at its truest,
is an act of love disguised as science.
When the journey ends,

or perhaps only changes form,
the air shimmers with unspoken goodbyes.
But grief, though heavy,
carries within it the seed of grace.

For love does not vanish with the body;
it migrates into memory, into light,
into every heart that dared to care.
A mother's tears water the ground of hope.

A father's touch,
seals a promise of forever.
A healer's hands, release what they once tried to hold,
trusting that the spirit finds its own horizon.

And in the quiet that follows,
one truth remains unshaken:
Love cannot be measured by weight or time,
nor confined to the cradle or the grave.

It endures, as the echo of a heartbeat felt in eternity,
as the breath that becomes wind,
as the light that continues to shine
long after the lamp is gone.

So let us remember, each life, however brief,
is a verse in the great hymn of creation.
Each caregiver, a witness to divinity.
Each parent, a poet of unconditional grace.

And every child, a teacher, radiant and pure,
who reminds us that in giving love,
We love beyond measure,
We become love. We become it.

Appendices

Appendix A — Clinical Tools: Supporting Bereavement and Compassionate Communication

This appendix provides practical tools for healthcare professionals and families navigating the emotionally profound journey of neonatal loss. Each resource aims to bridge science and soul, fostering communication, memory-making, and collective healing within the Neonatal Intensive Care Unit (NICU).

1. Bereavement Communication Guides

Purpose: To support clinicians and staff in approaching sensitive conversations with empathy, clarity, and respect.

Guiding Principles

- **Presence before words:** Begin by being fully present; silence can convey compassion when words fail.

- **Acknowledge the reality:** Use the baby's name; avoid euphemisms.

- **Listen actively:** Allow parents to express shock, guilt, or anger without interruption.

- **Balance hope and honesty:** Share medical realities compassionately while honoring emotional truths.

- **Follow up:** Compassion extends beyond the moment of loss—reach out in the days and weeks after.

Suggested Phrases

- "I am so sorry. Your baby is loved and will always be remembered."

- "We are here to walk this path with you."

- "Would you like to hold your baby or spend some quiet time together?"

- "Tell me about your baby—what name did you choose?"

Avoid

- Minimizing statements ("At least you have other children," "It wasn't meant to be").

- Technical jargon or detached medical explanations.

- Rushing the conversation to closure.

2. Memory-Making and Legacy Tools

Creating tangible memories can transform grief into enduring love. These practices affirm the sacredness of each life, no matter how brief.

Memory-Making Checklist

- **Hand and Footprints:** Ink or clay impressions, framed or included in a keepsake box.

- **Lock of Hair:** Collected with permission and sealed in a labeled envelope.

- **Photographs:** Professional or staff-taken photos in soft lighting, with parents' participation.

- **Personal Items:** Blanket, hat, or ID band placed in a remembrance box.

- **Name Certificate:** A personalized certificate affirming the baby's name, date of birth, and significance.

- **Memory Blanket or Quilt:** Option for families to contribute to a communal NICU remembrance project.

- **Spiritual Rituals:** Offer prayer, blessing, or candle-lighting according to the family's faith tradition.

Comfort Environment

- Dimmed lighting, privacy curtains, soft music, and supportive staff presence during memory-making.

- Offer tissues, water, and a gentle explanation of each step before proceeding.

3. Family Support and Resource Guide For Parents and Families

Immediate Support:

- Hospital chaplaincy or spiritual care services.

- Bereavement counselor or licensed therapist specializing in perinatal loss.

- Peer support groups for grieving parents.

- **Long-Term Healing:**

- Journaling prompts or remembrance ceremonies on anniversaries.

- Online support networks (e.g., *Share Pregnancy & Infant Loss Support, The Compassionate Friends*).

- Local community resources for grief and trauma recovery.

For Siblings and Extended Family

- Use age-appropriate explanations about death.

- Encourage artwork, storytelling, or writing letters to the baby.

- Offer family therapy if prolonged distress or guilt appears.

4. NICU Staff Support and Debriefing Tools

Purpose: To sustain emotional well-being, prevent burnout, and maintain compassionate resilience among healthcare providers.

Team Debrief Checklist

- Schedule a debrief after any neonatal loss.

- Encourage open reflection: What went well? What was difficult?

- Validate emotional responses—grief, sadness, guilt, or fatigue.

- Offer access to mental health professionals for ongoing support.

- Integrate mindfulness or compassion-based stress reduction (MBSR) practices for staff renewal.

Self-Care Reminders

- Take breaks between emotionally charged moments.

- Seek peer support; don't isolate.

- Remember: compassionate care includes caring for oneself.

5. Institutional and Educational Resources

Recommended References

- *National Perinatal Association Guidelines for Family-Centered Bereavement Care*

- *Resolve Through Sharing® Bereavement Training Program*

- *Perinatal Loss Guidelines — American College of Obstetricians and Gynecologists (ACOG)*

- *The Compassionate Friends Organization — www.compassionatefriends.org*

- *Share Pregnancy and Infant Loss Support — www.nationalshare.org*

6. Reflection for Caregivers

"Each life we touch leaves an imprint upon the soul of our practice. In every loss, we meet love in its purest form." *Arwin M. Valencia, MD*

Encourage journaling among NICU staff:

- *What moments have taught me the meaning of presence?*

- *How has this family's journey deepened my understanding of healing?*

- *What practices restore my sense of compassion and peace after loss?*

Appendix B — Scientific References

Research on Perinatal Loss, Stress Neurobiology, Compassion Science, and Grief Models

This appendix compiles key scientific and theoretical works that illuminate the physiological, psychological, and spiritual dimensions of perinatal loss and compassionate care. These references serve as foundational support for the integrative approach discussed throughout *Cradled in Light*—where evidence-based medicine meets the art of healing and human connection.

I. Perinatal Loss and Bereavement Research

Perinatal loss encompasses miscarriage, stillbirth, and neonatal death, each with profound psychological and social effects on parents and caregivers. Research continues to explore both the measurable health outcomes and the ineffable dimensions of parental grief.

Key References

1.   Cacciatore, J., & Bushfield, S. (2008). *Stillbirth: Embodied grief and the collapse of meaning.* Omega—Journal of Death and Dying, 56(2), 115–133.

2.   Kochen, E. M., Jenken, F., Boelen, P. A., & Smid, G. E. (2020). *Perinatal loss: Factors associated with*

parental grief trajectories. Journal of Psychosomatic Research, 133, 110111.

     3.   Fenstermacher, K., & Hupcey, J. (2013). *Perinatal bereavement: A principle-based concept analysis.* Journal of Advanced Nursing, 69(11), 2389–2400.

     4.   Gold, K. J., Leon, I., & Boggs, M. E. (2016). *Mental health outcomes in mothers after stillbirth: A review of the literature.* American Journal of Obstetrics & Gynecology, 215(4), 459–465.

     5.   Capitulo, K. L. (2005). *Perinatal grief online: Support for parents and health care providers.* MCN: The American Journal of Maternal/Child Nursing, 30(6), 389–395.

Notable Themes

- Parental identity continues despite loss ("continuing bonds" model).

- Grief outcomes improve with compassionate care and active memory-making.

- The importance of narrative medicine and ritual in meaning reconstruction.

II. Stress Neurobiology and the Psychophysiology of Grief

Understanding the neurobiological mechanisms of stress and attachment loss provides the medical foundation for compassionate care. The intersection of neuroscience, endocrinology, and psychology reveals how grief manifests in both body and mind.

Key References

1.   McEwen, B. S. (2007). *Physiology and neurobiology of stress and adaptation: Central role of the brain.* Physiological Reviews, 87(3), 873–904.

2.   Porges, S. W. (2011). *The Polyvagal Theory: Neurophysiological foundations of emotions, attachment, communication, and self-regulation.* W. W. Norton & Company.

3.   Hofer, M. A. (1994). *Hidden regulators in attachment, separation, and loss.* Monographs of the Society for Research in Child Development, 59(2–3), 192–207.

4.   Coan, J. A., & Sbarra, D. A. (2015). *Social baseline theory: The social regulation of risk and effort.* Current Opinion in Psychology, 1, 87–91.

5.   Schore, A. N. (2001). *Effects of a secure attachment relationship on right brain development, affect regulation, and infant mental health.* Infant Mental Health Journal, 22(1–2), 7–66.

Core Insights

- **Grief as a neurobiological stress response:** Involves limbic activation, cortisol dysregulation, and altered immune signaling.

- **Polyvagal safety:** Compassionate presence regulates autonomic arousal, promoting healing and emotional coherence.

- **Attachment disruption:** Loss in the perinatal period can rewire neural circuits related to safety and bonding.

III. Compassion Science and the Neurobiology of Care

Compassion is more than empathy—it is a biologically measurable and trainable prosocial response. Compassion science explores how neural and hormonal systems support caregiving and resilience in healthcare environments like the NICU.

Key References

1. Goetz, J. L., Keltner, D., & Simon-Thomas, E. (2010). *Compassion: An evolutionary analysis and empirical review.* Psychological Bulletin, 136(3), 351–374.

2. Klimecki, O. M., Leiberg, S., Lamm, C., & Singer, T. (2013). *Functional neural plasticity and associated*

changes in positive affect after compassion training. Cerebral Cortex, 23(7), 1552–1561.

3.   Doty, R. L. (2018). *Love and compassion: Neuroscientific perspectives.* Oxford University Press.

4.   Trzeciak, S., & Mazzarelli, A. J. (2019). *Compassionomics: The revolutionary scientific evidence that caring makes a difference.* Studer Group.

5.   Singer, T., & Bolz, M. (2012). *Compassion: Bridging practice and science.* Max Planck Institute.

Clinical Applications

- Compassion enhances patient outcomes and reduces clinician burnout.

- Neural correlates: activation of medial prefrontal cortex, anterior insula, and oxytocinergic pathways.

- Cultivating compassion through mindfulness, presence, and reflection creates physiological coherence and empathy resonance in NICU environments.

IV. Grief Models and Theories of Meaning-Making

The study of grief has evolved beyond stage models toward dynamic frameworks emphasizing adaptation, resilience, and continued bonds.

Key References

1.   Kübler-Ross, E. (1969). *On Death and Dying.* Macmillan.

2.   Worden, J. W. (2018). *Grief Counseling and Grief Therapy: A Handbook for the Mental Health Practitioner* (5th ed.). Springer Publishing.

3.   Stroebe, M., & Schut, H. (1999). *The Dual Process Model of coping with bereavement: Rationale and description.* Death Studies, 23(3), 197–224.

4.   Neimeyer, R. A. (2001). *Meaning reconstruction and the experience of loss.* American Psychological Association.

5.   Klass, D., Silverman, P. R., & Nickman, S. L. (Eds.). (1996). *Continuing Bonds: New understandings of grief.* Taylor & Francis.

6.   Bonanno, G. A. (2009). *The Other Side of Sadness: What the new science of bereavement tells us about life after loss.* Basic Books.

Conceptual Themes

- **Dual Process Model:** Grievers oscillate between loss-oriented and restoration-oriented coping.

- **Continuing Bonds:** Love endures beyond physical separation, redefining relationship rather than severing it.

- **Meaning Reconstruction:** Healing involves rewriting one's narrative of loss into a story of transformation.

- **Resilience Framework:** Many bereaved parents exhibit post-traumatic growth, particularly when supported by compassionate environments.

V. Integrative Perspectives: Bridging Science and Soul

Research increasingly supports an integrative model that unites clinical science, compassionate communication, and spiritual meaning.

Representative Works

1. Sulmasy, D. P. (2002). *A biopsychosocial-spiritual model for the care of patients at the end of life.* Gerontologist, 42(Special Issue 3), 24–33.

2. Puchalski, C. M. et al. (2014). *Improving the quality of spiritual care as a dimension of palliative care.* Journal of Palliative Medicine, 17(6), 642–656.

3.   Sinclair, S., et al. (2016). *Compassion in health care: An empirical model.* Journal of Pain and Symptom Management, 51(2), 193–203.

4.   Rushton, C. H. (2018). *Moral resilience: Transforming moral suffering in healthcare.* Oxford University Press.

5.   Attig, T. (2011). *How We Grieve: Relearning the World* (Revised ed.). Oxford University Press.

Emerging Synthesis

- Integrating neuroscience, spirituality, and compassion fosters a model of *whole-person care.*

- Empathy and mindful presence activate neural coherence and improve family-clinician communication.

- Meaning-making in grief becomes both a spiritual and neurobiological process, a restoration of inner coherence.

Conclusion

"Science describes the mechanisms of life; compassion gives them meaning. Healing begins when knowledge bows to love." *Maria Abrantes, MD*

This compendium reflects the evolving understanding that the journey through loss—both for families and clinicians—is as physiological as it is spiritual. Through evidence-based compassion, we transform suffering into sacred connection, bridging medicine and mystery in the healing continuum.

Appendix C — Reflection Journal

Prompts for Healthcare Professionals and Parents

The journey through love and loss in the Neonatal Intensive Care Unit (NICU) leaves indelible marks on both families and caregivers. Reflection allows these experiences to transform rather than traumatize—to become sources of meaning, empathy, and spiritual depth.

These journal prompts are designed as gentle invitations for dialogue with the self, the soul, and the sacred mystery of life.

Section I — For Parents and Families

Each prompt is crafted to help grieving parents honor their child's memory, process emotions, and rediscover light within the shadows of loss.

1. Honoring the Bond

- Describe the moment you first connected with your baby—before, during, or after birth.

- What emotions, sensations, or thoughts arise when you recall holding your baby or seeing them for the first time?

- How would you describe the love that continues to live between you and your child today?

2. The Healing Power of Memory

- What memories, objects, or rituals bring you comfort when you miss your baby?

- If you could write a letter to your baby, what would you say?

- How do you wish for your child's story to be remembered within your family?

3. Navigating the Seasons of Grief

- In what ways has grief changed over time for you?

- How do you care for yourself when the waves of sadness return unexpectedly?

- What does "healing" mean to you—not as forgetting, but as continuing to love?

4. Reconstructing Meaning

- What has this experience taught you about life, faith, or love?

- Have you discovered new strengths, insights, or sensitivities through this journey?

- If your baby could speak to you now, what message of peace or wisdom might they share?

5. Continuing Bonds and Legacy

- How do you keep your baby's presence alive in your daily life?

- Have you found ways to transform your grief into compassion for others?

- What would you like future parents going through similar loss to know or feel?

"Grief is love that has nowhere to go—until we give it form through remembrance." Arwin M. Valencia, MD

Section II — For Healthcare Professionals

The NICU is not only a place of medical miracles—it is a crucible for emotional and spiritual growth. Reflecting on these experiences nurtures compassion, integrity, and resilience in the healer's path.

1. Presence and Humanity

- Recall a moment when you felt profoundly connected to a family or infant. What made that moment sacred?

- How do you balance your professional role with your human heart when facing tragedy?

- When have silence and presence spoken louder than words?

2. Bearing Witness

- Describe a time when you were deeply moved by a family's love or strength.

- What emotions arise when caring for an infant at the threshold between life and death?

- How do you honor the babies who have touched your life and practice?

3. Compassion Fatigue and Renewal

- How does prolonged exposure to suffering affect your mind, body, and spirit?

- What practices help you return to center—breathing, prayer, nature, art, or connection?

- How can you create a small ritual to release emotional weight at the end of a difficult shift?

4. Meaning in Medicine

- Reflect on how your understanding of healing has evolved through your NICU experiences.

- How do you integrate scientific precision with compassionate presence?

- What values guide you when clinical outcomes cannot bring a cure, but love can still bring comfort?

5. The Call to Serve

- What inspired you to choose this profession— and how has it changed you?

- What do you believe your soul is learning through the work of caring for the most fragile lives?

- How do you wish to be remembered—not for what you did, but for how you cared?

"Healing begins the moment the clinician's heart synchronizes with the family's grief and love. In that resonance, science becomes sacred." **Maria Abrantes, MD, FAAP**

Section III — Shared Reflections: The Bridge Between Parent and Healer

These prompts invite dialogue and empathy between families and care teams, reminding both that compassion is reciprocal—that every story transforms everyone involved.

- What have we learned from each other about courage and tenderness?

- How does witnessing the other's pain deepen our understanding of love?

- What invisible threads connect all who enter the NICU—parent, child, and healer alike?

- How can gratitude become our shared language, even in loss?

- What light has emerged from the darkness, and how can it guide others forward?

Suggested Use

- **Parents:** Use these prompts as part of a remembrance journal or monthly reflection ritual.

- **Clinicians:** Integrate journaling into debrief sessions, mindfulness rounds, or reflective practice workshops.

- **Institutions:** Offer these pages as part of bereavement packets or wellness programs to foster connection and healing.

Section IV — Closing Meditation

In the stillness after the monitors quiet,

When only the heartbeat of memory remains,

Love continues—beyond fear, beyond form, beyond time.

May every tear become a seed of compassion.

May every life, however brief, become a spark of eternity.

A.M.V., M.D.

About the Author

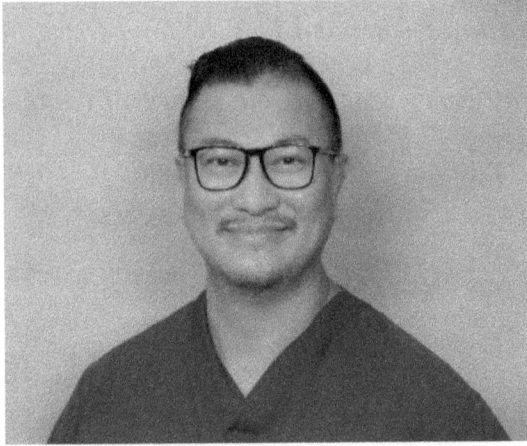

Arwin M. Valencia, MD, is a board-certified neonatologist whose career has been dedicated to caring for the most fragile beginnings of life. With decades of experience in neonatal intensive care, he blends the precision of medical science with the compassion of the human spirit, recognizing that healing extends far beyond physiology, it touches the soul.

Through his work, he has developed a holistic approach that integrates cutting-edge neonatal medicine with empathy, mindfulness, and spiritual awareness. His writings reflect this integration, exploring the sacred intersection of life, loss, and meaning within the walls of the NICU.

In *Cradled in Light*, he invites readers to witness the profound exchange between parent, child, and healer, a space where love becomes both medicine and memory, and where even the briefest lives illuminate eternity.

www.ingramcontent.com/pod-product-compliance
Lightning Source LLC
Chambersburg PA
CBHW031510270326
41930CB00006B/333